Color Atlas of
Pediatric Rheumatology

Barbara M. Ansell
Formerly Consultant Rheumatologist and Head of the Division of Rheumatology, Clinical Research Centre, Northwick Park Hospital, Harrow, England

Sue Rudge
Consultant Rheumatologist, Royal London Hospital and Queen Elizabeth Hospital for Children, Hackney, London, England

Jane G. Schaller
David and Leona Karp Professor and Chairman of Pediatrics, Tufts University, Medford, and Pediatrician-in-Chief, Floating Hospital for Infants and Children, Boston, Massachusetts, USA

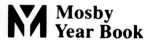
Mosby
Year Book

St. Louis   Baltimore   Boston   Chicago   London   Philadelphia   Sydney   Toronto

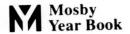
Mosby
Year Book

ISBN 0-8151-0221-6

English edition first published in 1992 by Wolfe Publishing Ltd,
2–16 Torrington Place, London WC1E 7LT, UK.

Library of Congress Cataloging-in-Publication Data

Ansell, Barbara M.
　　Color atlas of pediatric rheumatology / Barbara M. Ansell, Sue
Rudge, Jane G. Schaller.
　　　　p.　cm.
　　Includes bibliographical references and index.
　　ISBN 0-8151-0221-6
　　1. Rheumatism in children—Atlases.　　I. Rudge, Sue.
II. Schaller, Jane G., 1934–　　　III. Title.
　　[DNLM: 1. Rheumatic Diseases—in infancy & childhood—atlases.
WE 17 A618c]
RJ482.R48A56　1991
618.92′723–dc20
DNLM/DLC
for Library of Congress　　　　　　　　　　　91-19852
　　　　　　　　　　　　　　　　　　　　　　　　　　　CIP

CONTENTS

PREFACE

Not only is *paediatric rheumatology* a fledgling field, as noted in Chapter One, but indeed the field of rheumatology in general is a new one that barely spans 50 years. The rheumatic diseases are difficult to define *per se*: the term 'rheum' ('flux') itself has little meaning in modern language. However, these conditions share the property of chronic or recurrent inflammation of connective tissues of uncertain etiology. Since the musculoskeletal system is composed largely of connective tissue, arthritis and myositis are prominent components in the rheumatic diseases. Internal organs, such as the heart and lungs, may also be affected when their supporting connective tissues are inflamed. Since the connective tissues are so widely spread throughout the body, their inflammation can cause a myriad of symptoms and signs, which result in distinctly different patterns of disease. Although antecedent events are known for some of the rheumatic diseases, such as haemolytic streptococcal infections and rheumatic fever, basic causes and pathogenesis remain elusive. The variable symptoms and signs, the chronicity and recurrences, and the absence of curative therapy render the rheumatic diseases a challenge for the paediatrician and the rheumatologist alike. The scope of paediatric rheumatology is further increased by a host of non-rheumatic conditions that affect the musculoskeletal system or otherwise mimic rheumatic diseases, which must be identified before an appropriate diagnosis can be made. Childhood rheumatic diseases and the conditions that mimic them occupy a prominent place in paediatric practice. The chronicity and unpredictability of these illnesses and the long potential life span of affected children make their appropriate management – including early diagnosis – vital and challenging. Optimal care requires the input of a number of specialists – paediatric rheumatologists, physical and occupational therapists, orthopaedic surgeons, ophthalmologists, special care nurses, social workers, etc., all working as a team with the child's primary care physician.

Childhood rheumatic diseases differ in many ways from rheumatic diseases as they are seen in adults. In some instances the diseases seem to be different: for example, the subgroups of juvenile arthritis (JRA) differ from those of classic adult rheumatoid arthritis, except for seropositive disease. Some conditions seen in children, such as pauciarticular arthritis of young children and Kawasaki disease, are recognized rarely in adults, while some common adult conditions, such as gout, osteoarthritis, and polymyalgia rheumatica, are seen rarely or never in children. On a worldwide basis, rheumatic fever remains the most important of the childhood rheumatic diseases. In the US and UK, juvenile arthritis is the most common condition.

The mission of the authors is to illustrate the wide range of rheumatic disorders that affect children and those conditions that mimic them. We hope that this work will serve to instill in the student and practitioner alike an appreciation of the broad range of findings in these disorders, which will facilitate their proper recognition. We have included diagnostic guidelines for all of the conditions, utilizing accepted diagnostic or classification criteria where available. We do not discuss either laboratory studies or therapy in any detail, but concentrate on diagnosis and recognition.

We are grateful to all who have helped us, most especially to the many children from several continents and several decades who are portrayed here. We hope that continuing attention to these difficult and puzzling conditions will increase our knowledge of basic mechanisms and lead to better therapies and methods of prevention or cure, so that the burden of illness cast by rheumatic diseases will be lightened for the children of the future.

ACKNOWLEDGEMENTS

For the high standard of clinical photographs we are indebted to Mrs Jean Tyler at Wexham Park Hospital, Slough, Ms Annie Shields, Clinical Research Centre, Harrow, and Mr Simon Dove, Queen Elizabeth Hospital, Hackney, without whose expertise this book would not have been possible. We must also acknowledge the enormous help we have received from many, many colleagues.

In 1977 Eric Bywaters commented that 'Paediatric rheumatology is one of the latest arrivals among sub-specialties'. He felt that he could say he had seen it arrive, although he could not specify its birthday or place. The many who worked with him at Taplow felt that he certainly helped to rear 'this young child', and this book would not have been possible without his enthusiasm and ability to inspire others. We are also indebted to him for allowing us to use the slides of rheumatic fever and other rarities that he has collected during his long working life. The many years of assistance given by Ralph Wedgwood, another pioneer in paediatric rheumatology, are also gratefully acknowledged.

We would like to acknowledge our colleagues Dr Patricia Woo at the Clinical Research Centre, Harrow, Dr M. Ann Hall at Wexham Park Hospital, Slough, Dr M. Dillon at the Hospital for Sick Children, Great Ormond Street and Professor C. Wood at the Queen Elizabeth Hospital for Sick Children in Hackney. We would also like to acknowledge our colleagues at the University of Washington, the Children's Hospital in Seattle, and the Floating Hospital for Infants and Children in Boston for their generosity and assistance.

We are also very grateful to other colleagues for their willingness to refer patients and to allow us to use material so obtained. It is impossible to name all of them individually, but without them this collection could not have been achieved.

This work would also not have been possible without the cheerful help of Mrs Gerry Brown and Mrs Jenny Martin, who not only provided secretarial expertise, but were involved in obtaining slides for copying and contacting colleagues for their permission to use referred patients.

HISTORICAL SUMMARY

The first description of a case of juvenile arthritis was given by Cornil in 1864, and in 1871 Lewis-Smith from New York reported on a child of 3 years who had suffered a febrile onset at the age of 9 months. Pictorial evidence was seen in Robert Adam's book on *Rheumatic Gout* in 1873, and in Alfred Baring Garrod's book *Gout and Rheumatic Gout* in 1876. Charles West, who founded the Great Ormond Street Hospital for Sick Children in London, in some of his later *Lectures on the Diseases of Infancy and Childhood* gave some four paragraphs regarding chronic arthritis in children, which he considered a rare occurrence. Numerous French authors were describing cases, including small series, but it was George Frederic Still who in 1896 gave a full description of the disease and even attempted a taxonomic classification, based on seeing 19 cases and reviewing the notes of three others during his two-year residency at Great Ormond Street. Following this, in Great Britain chronic arthritis in children was referred to as Still's disease (Bywaters, 1977).

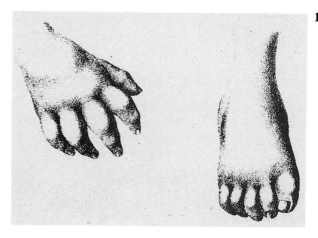

1 Illustration of chronic polyarthritis in a child, from Alfred Baring Garrod, *Gout and Rheumatic Gout*, 1876. (Courtesy of E.G.L. Bywaters and *Arthritis & Rheumatism*, 1977.)

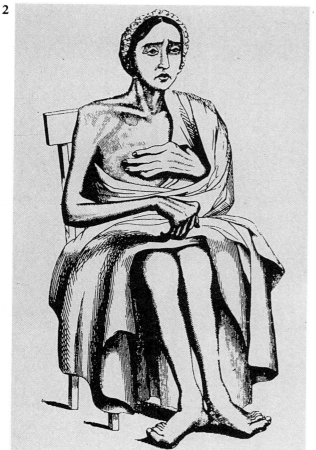

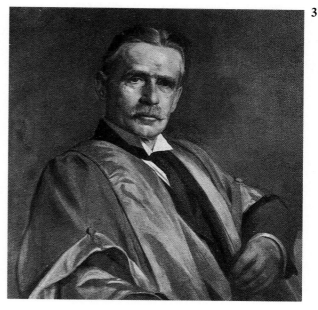

2 Margaret Burgess at 27 years of age, who suffered onset of arthritis at age 13, from Robert Adams, *Rheumatic Gout*, 1873. (Courtesy of E.G.L. Bywaters and *Arthritis & Rheumatism*, 1977.)

3 Copy of the portrait of George Frederic Still, the first Professor of Paediatrics at King's College Hospital, London. The portrait now hangs in their boardroom. (Courtesy of Dr Eric Hamilton, UK.)

During the early part of the twentieth century the advancing front in paediatric rheumatology was rheumatic fever and the incrimination of group A beta haemolytic streptococcus in its etiology. Despite a declining incidence since the 1890s, when Eric Bywaters started the Rheumatic Research Unit for juveniles at the Canadian Red Cross Memorial Hospital, Taplow, in 1947 rheumatic fever was still a major problem, and all except four of its 100 beds were occupied by children with rheumatic fever. By the 1950s, in the developed countries rheumatic fever was decreasing rapidly, and new investigations – the lupus erythematosus (LE) cell phenomenon and Rose–Waaler tests – together with the develop-ment of cortisone were associated with an upsurge of interest in chronic arthritis, which at Taplow was particularly concerned with that in childhood. A similar interest was also starting to occur in many other countries: notably the USA, Scandinavia and at Garmisch Parten Kirchen in Germany. The Taplow Unit served as a rendezvous for people interested in chronic arthritis and particularly that of childhood. Many notables visited the unit, including one of the co-authors of this book, who spent a sabbatical there, during which time she correlated the high incidence of antinuclear antibodies widely reported in juvenile chronic arthritis with chronic iridocyclitis in pauci-articular onset patients.

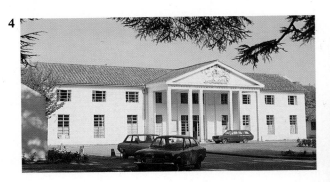

4 The imposing front entrance of the Canadian Red Cross Memorial Hospital, Taplow, which was the home of the Juvenile Rheumatism Unit, later to become the Medical Research Council Rheumatism Unit.

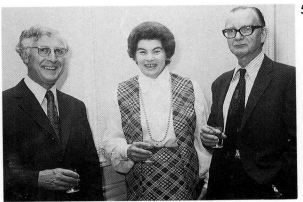

5 Ken Smiley (ophthalmic surgeon), Barbara M. Ansell (rheumatologist) and Eric Bywaters.

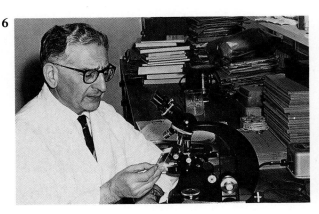

6 L.E. Glynn, who was Deputy Director at the Rheumatism Unit at Taplow, and in charge of the research laboratories.

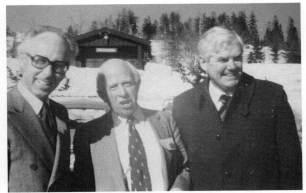

7 George Arden (centre), who is an orthopaedic surgeon of the Windsor group and was the first orthopaedic surgeon to be closely associated with the unit; seen here with Norbet Schwend (Switzerland) and Jan Pahle (Norway) at the workshop in Oslo in 1977.

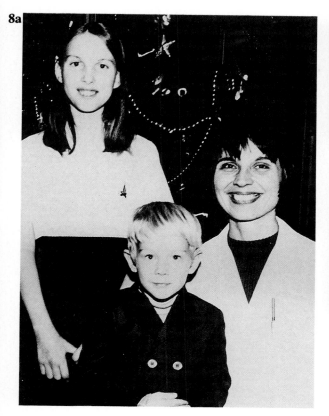

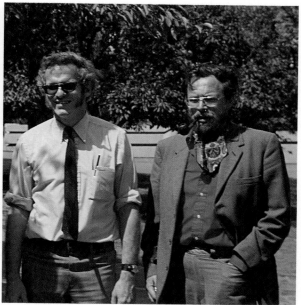

8a Jane Schaller with patients in Seattle in 1970, and **8b** Roger Hollister and Ralph Wedgewood, also in Seattle, in 1973.

The meeting that Jane Schaller and Virgil Hanson organized in Park City, USA, in 1976 brought together people from various specialities who were working in or might have had a peripheral interest in paediatric rheumatology, in order to focus attention on and suggest new directions in this field. Not only did this produce a major supplement publication in *Arthritis and Rheumatism*, which gathered together information then available, but it also stimulated the idea of regional arthritis resources being mobilized, and of the further development of the paediatric Rheumatology Collaborative Study groups for the progressive assessment of new drugs in the management of such children. A year later, in 1977, the late Eimar Munthe, under the auspices of the European League Against Rheumatism (EULAR), organized a workshop on the care of children with chronic arthritis. Out of this a working party, which subsequently became a full EULAR committee, grew to further the interest in paediatric rheumatology throughout Europe. This it certainly has done, predominantly at the clinical level; but it is now planning collaborative studies. These workshops coincided with Professor Bywaters' retirement and

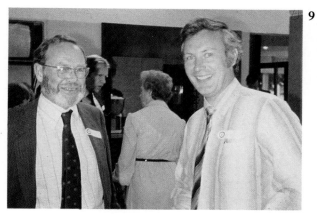

9

9 John Keen, a paediatrician at Manchester (the first to be associated with a regional clinic) and John Sills, a paediatrician at Liverpool (who is presently chairman of the British Paediatric Rheumatology Group) comparing notes at a meeting in 1983 at Fulmer Lodge, where the need for and planning of regional services, and the problems of caring for the chronic child at home and in the community, were discussed in full.

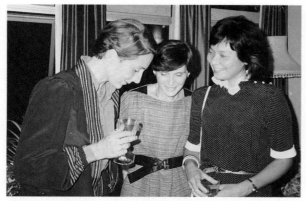

10 A social group after the British Society of Rheumatology (BSR) Course at the Clinical Research Centre, Harrow, in 1986, showing Gabriella Lenti from Italy, Guanida Kerimovic from Yugoslavia and Pat Woo, presently Head of Molecular Rheumatology at the Clinical Research Centre.

the transfer of the Medical Research Council Rheumatism Unit to the Clinical Research Centre at Northwick Park Hospital, Harrow, England. It was at this time that regional treatment facilities for children in Great Britain developed, starting with Manchester, and followed rapidly by Leeds, Newcastle and Scotland; over the last decade a number of new centres have been set up by interested doctors. Such doctors meet regularly through the Rheumatology Group of the British Paediatric Association and British Society of Rheumatology, when sessions are set aside for reviews, presentation of new work and general discussions. In Europe there is an annual meeting of paediatric rheumatologists under the auspices of EULAR, while the American College of Rheumatology and the American Academy of Pediatrics provide a similar background for the USA and Canada.

JUVENILE CHRONIC (RHEUMATOID) ARTHRITIS

Definition:
- A chronic arthritis that persists for a minimum of six consecutive weeks in one or more joints, commencing before the age of 16 years and after active exclusion of other causes (Cassidy *et al.*, 1989; Ansell, 1990)

Classification:
- By mode of onset during the first six months (Cassidy *et al.*, 1989; Prieur *et al.*, 1990)

Systemic disease:
- High remittent fever with one or more of the following – rash, hepatomegaly, splenomegaly, generalized lymphadenopathy, serositis, usually pericarditis
- Arthritis may be absent at the onset, but myalgia or arthralgia are usually present

Polyarthritic onset:
- Five or more joints develop in the onset period – usually somewhat insidiously and symmetrically
- May be further divided by the presence of IgM rheumatoid factor

Pauci-articular onset:
- The commonest mode with four or fewer joints involved, particularly knees and ankles
- Two clear subgroups have emerged, notably young children with positive antinuclear antibodies who are at risk from chronic iridocyclitis, and older boys (aged 9 upwards) who frequently carry the histocompatible leucocyte antigen (HLA) B27
- Others presenting in this way include juvenile psoriatic arthritis, the arthritis of inflammatory bowel disease and Reiter's syndrome, while some are as yet unclassified

Systemic Onset Disease

General characteristics:
- Usually begins before 5 years of age, but can occur throughout childhood into adult life
- Equal in boys and girls less than 5 years old; female predominance in those over 5 years old

Clinical features:
- High remittent fever
- Myalgia
- Arthralgia
- Malaise
- Rash – salmon pink or red maculopapular eruption
- Lymphadenopathy – cervical, epitrochlear, axillary and inguinal
- Hepatosplenomegaly
- Serositis – particularly pericarditis
- Hepatitis
- Progressive anaemia
- Disseminated intravascular coagulation
- Arthritis – knees, wrists and carpi, ankles and tarsi, neck, followed by other joints

Investigations:
- Erythrocyte sedimentation rate (ESR) – high
- Haemoglobin ↓
- White blood cell count ↑ (neutrophil leucocytosis)

Investigations (*cont.*):
- Platelets – raised
- IgM rheumatoid factor – negative
- Antinuclear antibodies (ANA) – negative

Course and prognosis:
- Half will have recurrent episodes of systemic disease
- Progressive arthritis occurs in about a third, irrespective of whether there are systemic exacerbations
- The younger the age of onset, the greater the risk of poor growth, both somatic and joints
- Amyloidosis occurs in some children with persistent disease activity, predominantly among Europeans

Management:
- Splinting to prevent deformity
- Physiotherapy to maintain joint mobility and muscle function
- Non-steroidal anti-inflammatory drugs (NSAID) to control pain, inflammation and fever
- Corticosteroids in severe disease, either as a single daily dose or given on alternate days
- Slow-acting drugs are of questionable benefit and may be dangerous during systemic disease

11

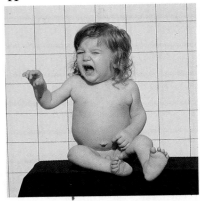

11 This 11-month-old developed a high fever followed by massive lymphadenopathy, irritability and, later, the maculopapular rash of systemic juvenile chronic arthritis (JCA).

12 This 3-year-old boy developed persistent fever following a sore throat, which was associated with the development of limb pain followed by swelling. On examination he was found to have widespread lymphadenopathy and marked hepatosplenomegaly.

12

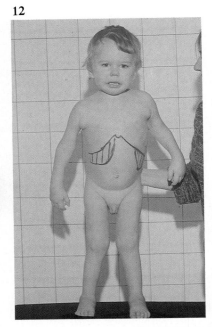

13

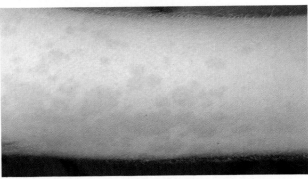
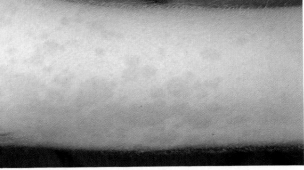

13 A typical swinging fever chart.

14 A maculopapular eruption, slightly raised at the height of the fever, in a 7-year-old Caucasian boy.

14

15

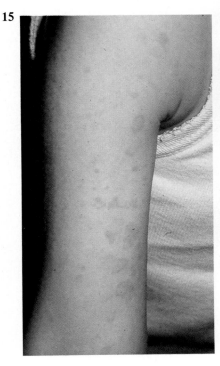

16

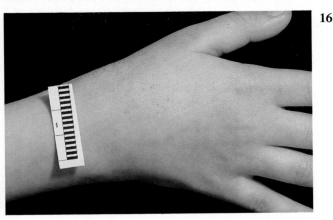

15 Similar rash on the inner aspect of the arm in a 5-year-old Indian boy; note the characteristic central pallor in some lesions.

16 Systemic onset JCA with swelling over the wrist and extending over the carpus, and a typical rash in a 7-year-old Caucasian girl.

17 Massive pericardial effusion in a 5-year-old girl who presented with a typical swinging fever, an occasional maculopapular rash and arthralgia. There had been little complaint of chest pain, but she was noted to have some difficulty in breathing and a slight rise in her jugular venous pressure.

18 A girl with liver enlargement and dysfunction early in her systemic illness.

19, 20 Systemic onset at age 3 years, followed by a polyarthritis that, within 4 months, was affecting her neck, shoulders, elbows, wrists, hips and ankles. The lateral view (**20**) shows the contractures.

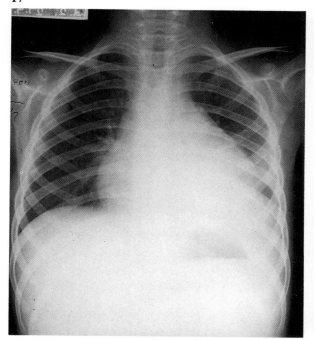

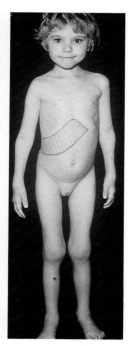

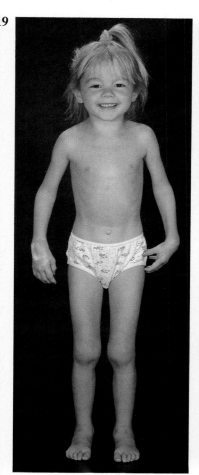

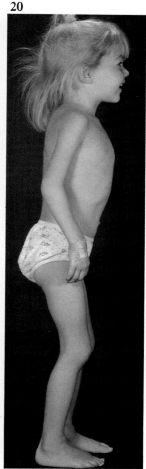

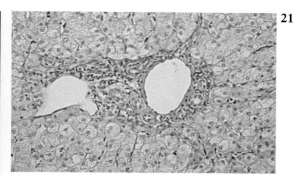

21 Liver biopsy from a 5-year-old boy who presented with high spiking fevers, massive hepatosplenomegaly, pleuritis, leucocytosis, and weight loss. Laboratory studies revealed leucocytosis, mildly elevated serum transaminase and bilirubin levels, and negative viral studies. The liver histology shows periportal collections of inflammatory cells, chiefly mature lymphocytes; scattered inflammatory cells are also present in the sinusoids (H & E preparation, × 75). A typical polyarthritis and rheumatoid rash began later, enabling a diagnosis of systemic onset JRA. His liver disease improved as his systemic disease regressed, but severe destructive arthritis developed.

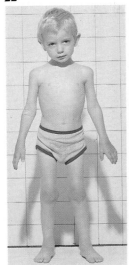
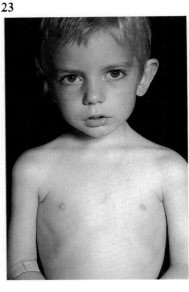

22 This 5-year-old boy presented with fever, rash and neck pain, and was initially thought to have meningitis. Note the torticollis, slight loss of full movement of the elbows, straight wrists, and swelling of the knees and ankles.

23 Close-up of the patient shown in **22**, some 3 months later. Note the persistent torticollis, his facial expression of misery, and swelling of both shoulders. The rash is still present.

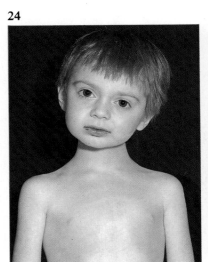
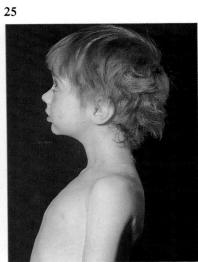
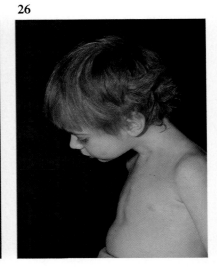

24 High fever with general malaise and persistent torticollis.

25, 26 Loss of extension, but some flexion, in the same patient as in **24**.

27 X-ray of subluxation of C_2 on C_3, in the same patient as in **24**. He was gently manipulated into a neutral position under the image intensifier. Following immobilization in a collar he suffered no further problems.

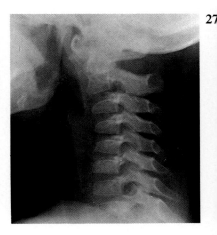

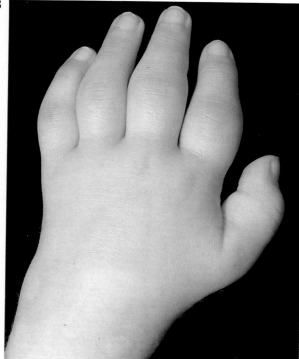

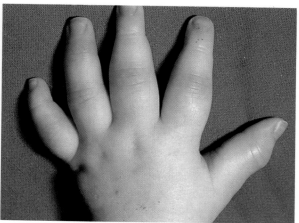

29 Very acute swelling of proximal interphalangeal joints in an 18-month-old, 9 weeks after presentation with fever.

28 Acute swelling of wrist, carpus and, particularly, proximal interphalangeal joints, including the terminal interphalangeal joints, which are reddened and associated with marked thickening of the flexor tendon. Note also the terminal interphalangeal joint involvement on the third and fourth finger in this boy aged 3 who had presented as a pyrexia of unknown origin (PUO) 6 weeks earlier.

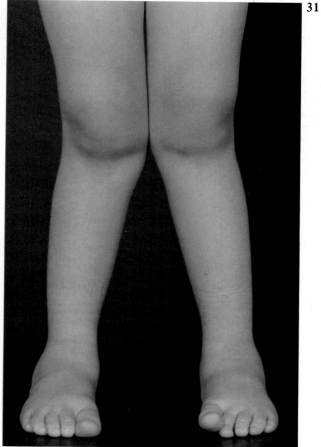

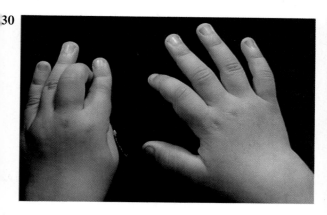

30 Some 18 months after presentation with a pericardial effusion, this boy shows: soft-tissue swelling of the wrists and carpi, which are tending to sublux; soft-tissue swelling of the metacarpophalangeal joints, particularly the left; and flexor tenosynovitis, causing contracture of the left middle finger.

31 The same patient as in **30**, showing persistent arthritis of the knees, with valgus deformity that developed over the preceding 12 months. Note that he also has involvement of both ankles and great toes.

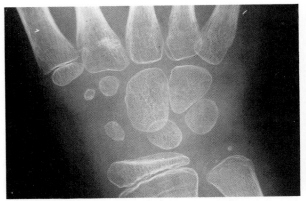

32 Systemic onset occurred 1 year previously in this 7-year-old, followed by persistent wrist synovitis.

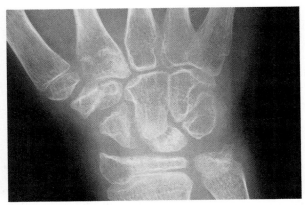

33 Same patient as in 32, 2 years later. There is angulation and overgrowth of all the carpal bones, with commencing bony fusion at the base of the second metacarpal to the carpus.

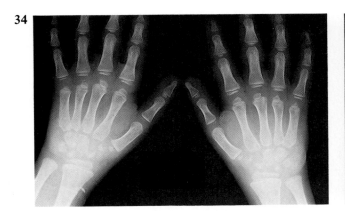

34 Systemic onset occurred 6 years previously, at 18 months of age, with synovitis unremitting from the third month of illness. Note the extensive radiocarpal and carpal changes, together with the widening of the phalanges due to periosteal accretion. Metacarpal epiphyses are showing early squaring.

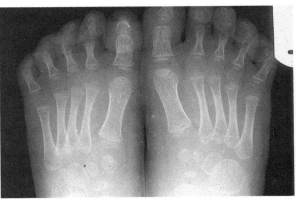

35 Foot X-ray 5 years after systemic onset and with persisting disease activity. Note the changes in the tarsal bones, with osteoporosis and widening of the forefoot and commencing irregular ossification of the metatarsal head.

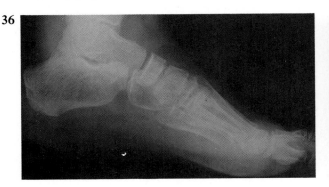

36 Lateral foot X-ray of a child 5 years after onset, with some squaring of the navicula and minor alteration in alignment of the talus and calcaneum. The disease is now inactive.

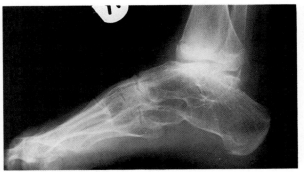

37 Lateral foot X-ray 8 years after systemic onset with persistent disease activity. Note the bony fusion of the talus with navicula and calcaneum, and bony fusion of the other tarsal bones.

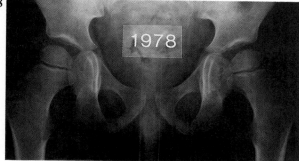

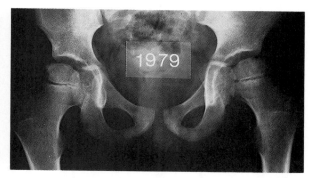

38–40 Sequential X-rays of the hips in a boy who had suffered a systemic onset some 18 months before the first X-ray was taken, and had required high-dose corticosteroid therapy because of severe pericardial problems. **38** shows early lateral subluxation with minimal change in the shape of the femoral heads. One year later (**39**), changes to the femoral head have increased and anteversion is more obvious. Two years further into the disease (**40**), there is acetabular irregularity, narrowing of joint space, increased abnormality of the femoral heads, persistent anteversion and large lesser trochanters.

40

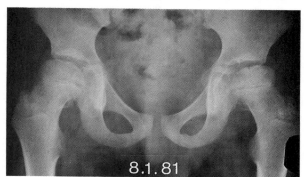

41

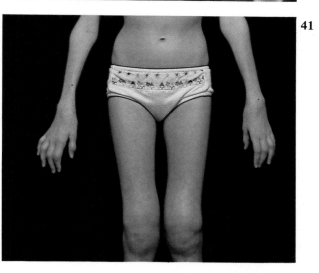

41 Onset of systemic disease at age 9. Persistent arthritis with marked boggy swelling around the elbows, wrists and knees.

42 Arthrogram of left elbow of patient in **41**, showing extensive size of the cavity with thickening around the radial head.

43 Shoulder cyst 6 months after systemic onset in association with arthritis of the knees, ankles, hips and wrists in a 7-year-old girl.

42

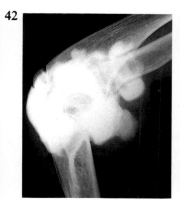
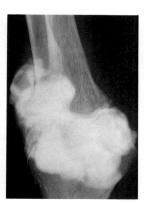

43

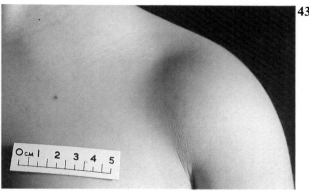

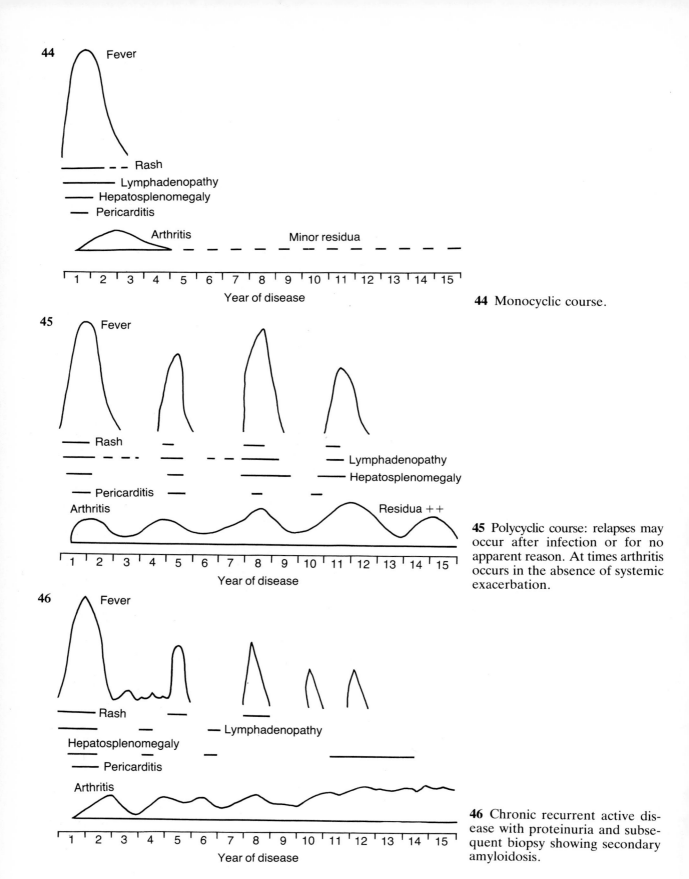

44 Monocyclic course.

45 Polycyclic course: relapses may occur after infection or for no apparent reason. At times arthritis occurs in the absence of systemic exacerbation.

46 Chronic recurrent active disease with proteinuria and subsequent biopsy showing secondary amyloidosis.

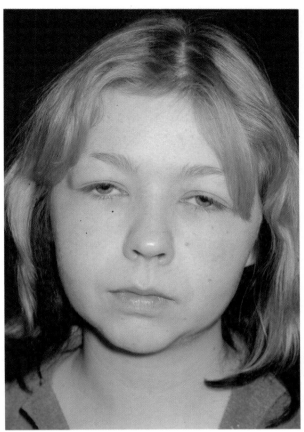

47 Oedema of the face due to amyloidosis causing a nephrotic syndrome. This has been known to develop as quickly as within 1 year, but it usually takes a minimum of 5 years in the presence of active disease.

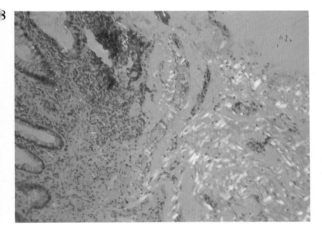

48 Rectal biopsy stained with congo red, amyloidoses is shown on apple green birefringence under polarized light.

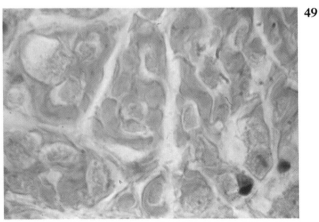

49 Cardiac amyloid in a patient who went into progressive heart failure and died.

Polyarthritic Onset: IgM Rheumatoid Factor Negative

General characteristics:
- Any age, occasionally before the first birthday
- Female predominance

Clinical features:
- Polyarthritis can affect any joint; the most commonly affected are the knees, wrists, ankles and proximal and distal interphalangeal joints of the hands; metacarpophalangeal joints are often spared
- Limitation of neck and temporomandibular movement is common
- Flexor tenosynovitis
- Low-grade fever, occasionally
- Mild lymphadenopathy and hepatosplenomegaly, occasionally.

Investigations:
- ESR – elevated
- Haemoglobin – may be reduced

Investigations (*cont.*):
- White blood count – mild neutrophil leucocytosis
- Platelets – moderate thrombocytosis
- IgM rheumatoid factor – negative
- ANA – occasionally positive

Course and prognosis:
- Variable
- May be monocyclic but prolonged over several years with good functional outcome
- Recurrent episodes tend to cause progressive deformities

Management:
- Splinting to prevent deformity
- Physiotherapy to maintain and improve joint and muscle function
- NSAIDs to control pain and inflammation
- Slow-acting drugs should be considered if there is progressive deformity

50

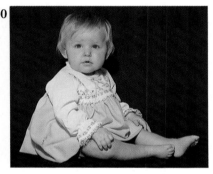

50 This girl developed swelling of both knees at about 6 months old, which steadily increased; note that the knees are taking up a position of flexion. Other joints, notably the ankles, fingers and wrist, have become involved.

51 This 2½-year-old girl had an acute onset of widespread prolific synovitis, affecting the knees and ankles, wrists, elbows and fingers. Her knees are already starting to sublux.

52 This 5-year-old girl presented with swelling of knees, ankles and elbows. Flexion contractures of the knees cause her to stand with flexion deformity at both hips; neither elbow extends fully, and she has severe wrist synovitis. Her neck is thrust slightly forward and is limited in movement.

51

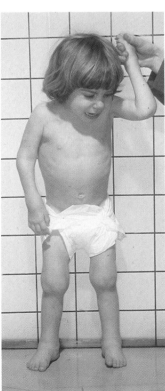

52

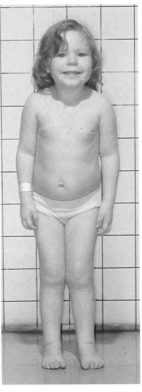

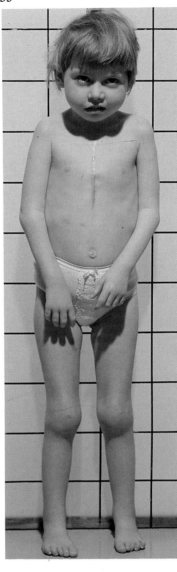

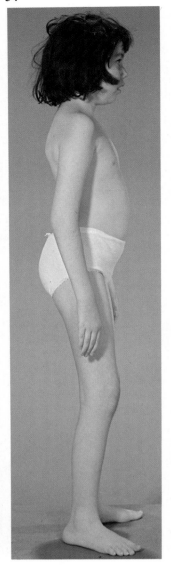

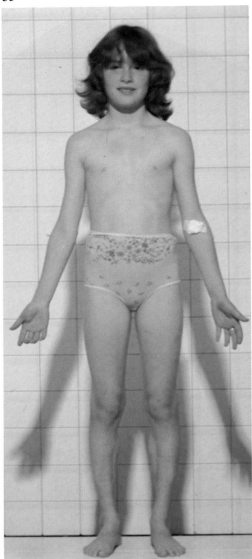

53 This girl, now aged 6, had little evidence of overt synovitis, and no complaints; but functionally she slowly deteriorated and had developed contractures at elbows, wrists, hips and knees, and stands with a poor posture and with inversion of her feet.

54 Lateral view of a 10-year-old who also presented with a general stiffening of joints over a 1-year period. Note the poked forward shoulder, loss of extension of the elbows, and flexed hips and knees.

55 This 11-year-old presented with pain, particularly in the knees and hands and, to a lesser extent, the ankles. She looks normal, but on palpation there was a soft-tissue swelling of the joints, about which she was complaining.

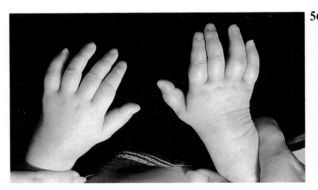

56 Slight swelling of the wrist and severe swelling of the fingers with early flexion contractures in a 7-month-old girl.

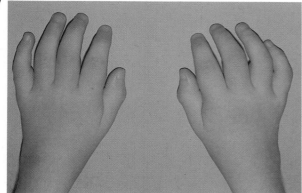

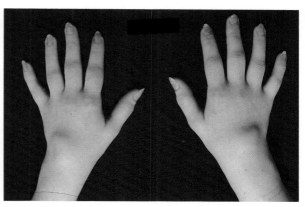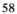

57 This 18-month-old shows soft-tissue swelling of the wrists, with a tendency to hyperextension at the metacarpophalangeal joints, and flexion deformities commencing in all the proximal interphalangeal joints with marked flexor tenosynovitis.

58 This girl, aged 6, presented with dorsal sheath swelling, associated with loss of movement at the wrists, and slight swelling of the metacarpophalangeal joints 2 and 3, but marked swelling of the proximal interphalangeal joints, which are beginning to flex.

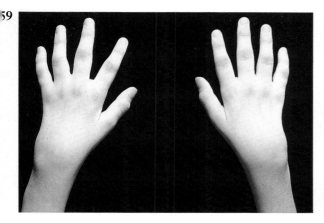
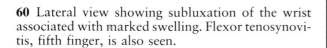

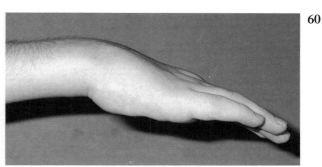

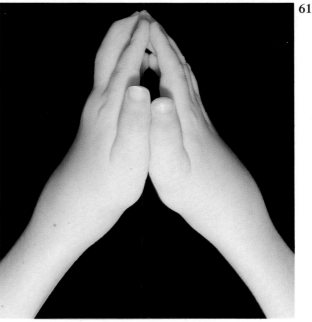

59 Marked swelling over the dorsum of the hand in a girl aged 11 years; there is only slight finger involvement.

60 Lateral view showing subluxation of the wrist associated with marked swelling. Flexor tenosynovitis, fifth finger, is also seen.

61 Lateral view in a boy aged 9 who had marked soft-tissue swelling of the wrist, with subluxation and some involvement of the finger joints. Thumb interphalangeal joint involvement is obvious in this view.

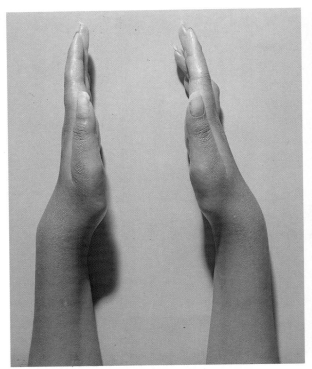

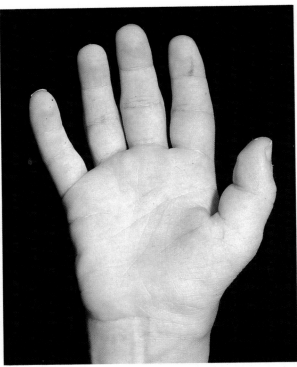

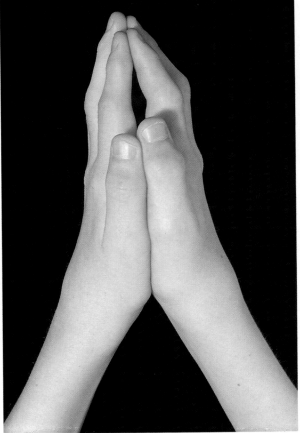

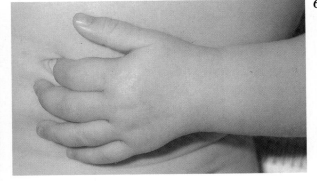

62 Lateral view of both wrists, showing soft-tissue swelling and subluxation, in a 10-year-old Kuwaiti girl with a disease of 11 months' duration.

63 Marked swelling of the flexor tendons affecting the thumb and all the fingers.

64 Lateral view of an 11-year-old's hands with one year's history showing soft-tissue swelling of the wrists, which have maintained a reasonable position, but early flexion contractures of the fingers, with involvement of the flexor tendons and proximal interphalangeal joints. Again, marked swelling of the interphalangeal joints of both thumbs is seen.

65 Marked soft-tissue swelling of the flexor tendons and proximal interphalangeal joints in a baby.

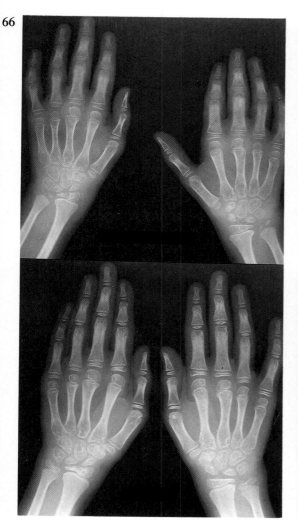

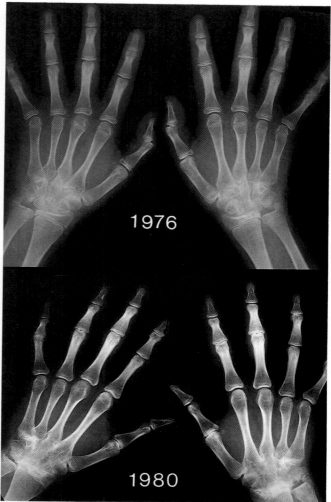

66 X-ray, 1 year after onset, shows crowding and overgrowth of the carpal bones and soft-tissue swelling around the metacarpophalangeal and proximal interphalangeal joints, with juxta articular osteoporosis. After 2 years, with reduction of disease activity, there has been overall growth of the hand, straightening of the fingers and improvement of the osteoporosis. The carpi have shown some further change with crowding.

67 This 11-year-old had carpal changes 9 months from onset. After 4 years, there is bony fusion of the carpus onto the metacarpals and a narrowing of the proximal interphalangeal joint spaces.

68 **69**

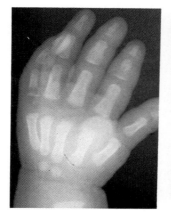

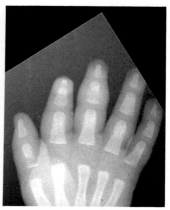

68, 69 These X-rays of a hand of an 8-month-old with severe finger involvement show marked soft-tissue swelling due to flexor tendon involvement, but no bony changes.

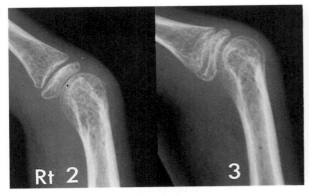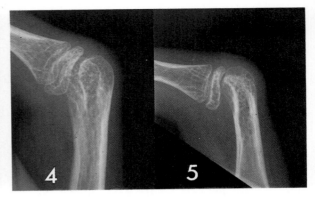

70 Lateral view of proximal interphalangeal joints in an 11-year-old boy with severe boutonnière deformity.

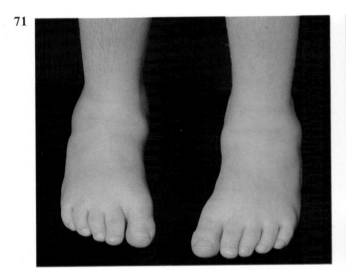

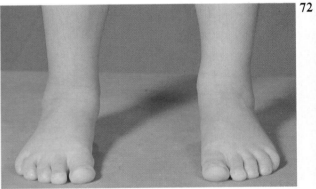

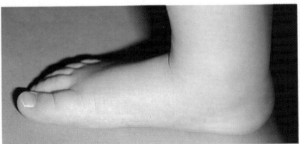

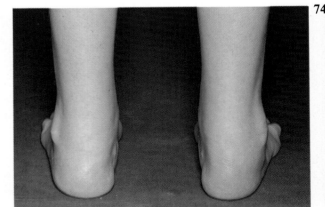

71 Soft-tissue swelling of both ankles, the right a little worse than the left. The right foot is already taking up a slightly varus position, extra pressure being thrown on the right great toe.

72 More proliferative synovitis around the ankles with more pronounced varus forefoot deformity with enlargement of the first metatarsophalangeal joint. Note the marked swelling extending over the dorsum of the foot to the first ray.

73 This 2-year-old half-Chinese girl has general fullness around the ankle and tendo Achilles.

74 Posterior view of a girl with ankle and hind foot involvement. Note the thickening around the tendo Achilles.

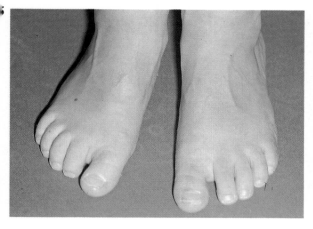

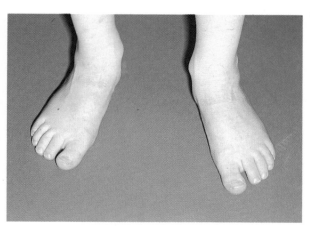

75 This boy has soft-tissue swelling of the ankle, general fullness over the tarsus, and early clawing of the toes.

76 After 3 years, the boy in **75** has marked valgus deformity at the ankles with severe hind foot involvement. There has been a slight discrepancy in growth, since one foot is not as large as the other.

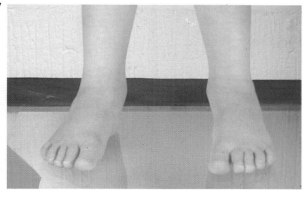

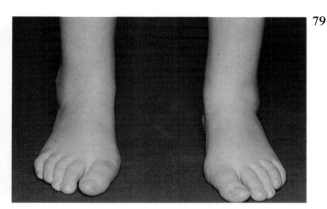

77, 78 This child, with 1 year's disease, shows marked valgus deformity commencing in the hind foot. Note from the sole of the foot (**78**) that weight bearing is predominantly on the heels and the first metatarsophalangeal joint.

79 This child, with ankle swelling, also has severe forefoot involvement, causing lateral deviation with early hallux valgus of the great toes and clawing of the metatarsophalangeal joints, with some soft-tissue swelling over the metatarsophalangeal joints.

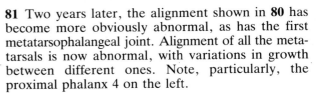

80 X-ray after 1 year of foot involvement showing a slight change in alignment of the first great toe.

81 Two years later, the alignment shown in **80** has become more obviously abnormal, as has the first metatarsophalangeal joint. Alignment of all the metatarsals is now abnormal, with variations in growth between different ones. Note, particularly, the proximal phalanx 4 on the left.

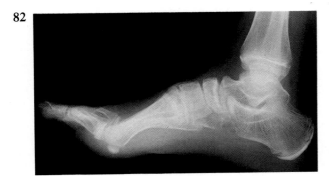

82 Lateral foot X-ray showing the narrowing of the talonavicular joint space and upward movement of the navicular, causing a pseudo pes cavus deformity.

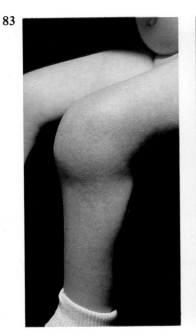

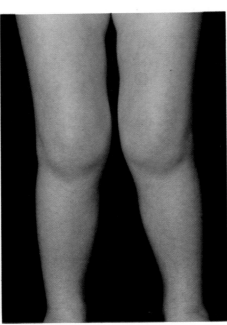

83 Marked soft-tissue swelling with effusion in the knee of a girl of 11 months who refused to straighten her legs.

84 Soft-tissue swelling of about 2 months' duration of both knees in a 3-year-old; note the tendency to valgus deformity and subluxation.

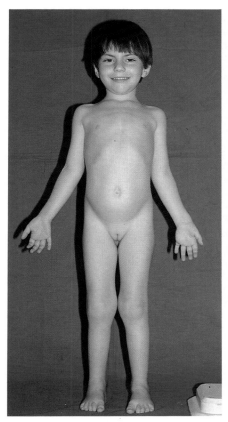

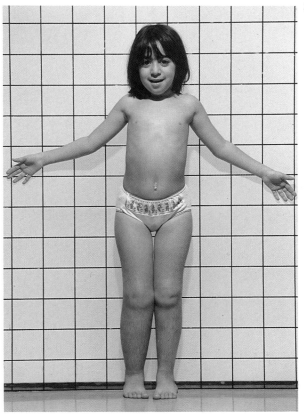

85 This 6-year-old girl has marked swelling of both knees and both elbows, and some involvement of the ankles and wrists.

86 Generalized polyarthritis, with particular swelling of the knees. Lymphoedema, seen here in the right leg, is an occasional complication of severe knee synovitis.

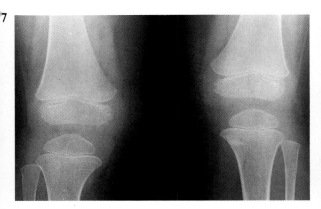

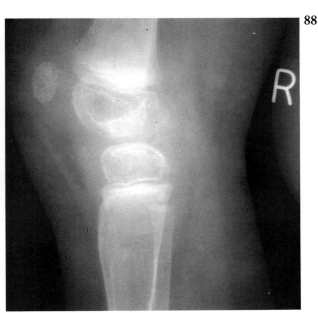

87 X-rays of knees 6 months after onset in a 3-year-old. Note the slight irregularity in epiphyses, but no other abnormality.

88 Lateral X-ray of a knee showing severe osteoporosis, subluxation of the tibia, and early overgrowth and irregularities of the patella.

89

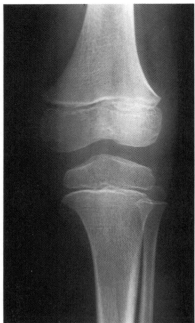

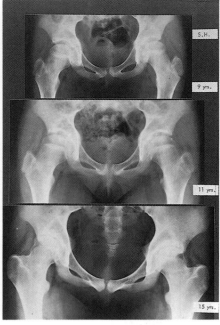

90

89 X-ray of a knee in a 9-year-old with soft-tissue swelling of 1 year's duration. Note the widening of the intercondylar notch of the femoral epiphysis.

90 Hip changes 1 year from onset; at the age of 9 years there was loss of joint space, which progressed over the next 2 years with early acetabular change; 4 years later there was early protrusion, reduction of joint space, and irregularity of the femoral head.

91

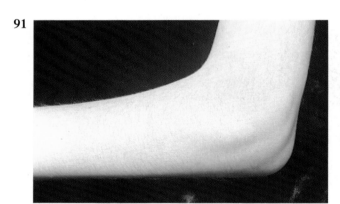

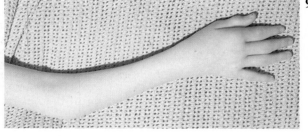

92

91 Close-up of swelling of an elbow. Note the pad of soft-tissue swelling over the radial head (*see* **42**).

92 Difficulty in extending the elbow in a boy with polyarthritis. Note the moderately severe involvement of the wrists and joints of the hand.

93

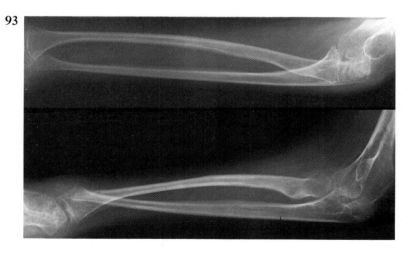

93 X-ray of elbows and forearms showing differential growth of the radius and ulna some 5 years into the disease. Marked growth changes are present in elbow epiphyses.

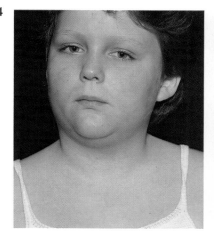

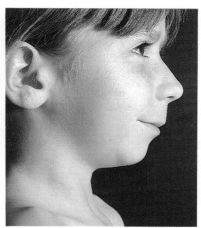

94 Torticollis due to involvement of the cervical spine.

95 Underdevelopment of the jaw in a 5-year-old who has poor growth in the neck.

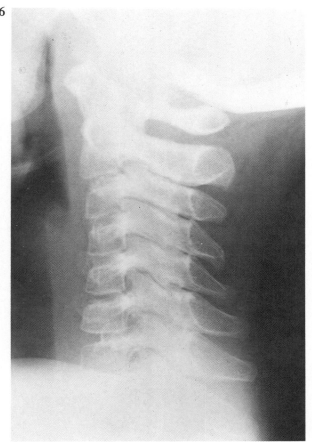

96 Lateral X-ray of cervical spine showing loss of normal curve, variation in size of vertebrae and narrowing of apophyseal joint spaces.

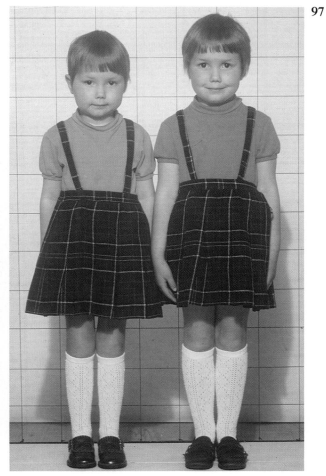

97 The identical twin on the left developed polyarthritis at the age of 2½ years; here, 3 years later, without ever having had corticosteroids, she is generally smaller than her twin. This shows the overall impairment of growth associated with continuing disease activity. Concordance of the disease is uncommon.

Polyarthritic Onset, IgM Rheumatoid Factor Positive

General characteristics:
- Over 8 years of age at onset
- Female predominance

Clinical features:
- Polyarthritis affecting any joint, but particularly the small joints of the wrists, hands, ankles, and feet; knees and hips often early, with elbows and other joints later
- Rheumatoid nodules on pressure points, particularly elbows
- Vasculitis – uncommon and often late, nail fold lesions, ulceration.

Investigations:
- ESR – usually elevated
- Haemoglobin – moderate anaemia
- IgM rheumatoid factor – persistently positive and in high titre
- ANA – may be positive

Investigations (*cont.*):
- HLA DR4 – frequently present
- Radiographically – early erosive changes of affected joints, particularly of hands and feet

Course and prognosis:
- Persistent activity with serious joint destruction and poor functional outcome
- Additional long-term hazards include atlanto-axial subluxation, aortic incompetence, and amyloidosis

Management:
- Splinting to preserve function
- Physiotherapy to maintain and improve joint and muscle function
- NSAIDs
- Slow-acting drugs early (months)
- Methotrexate
- Surgical intervention, such as replacement arthroplasties, often required later

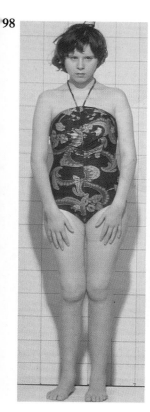

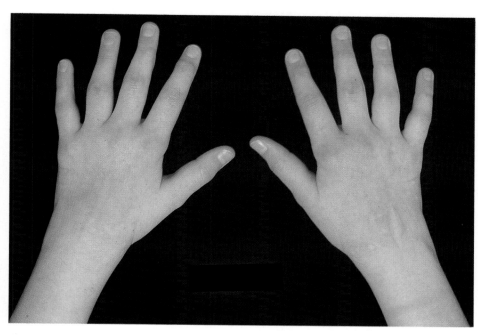

98 Adolescent girl presenting with pain and stiffness in the feet, particularly on rising, followed by the hands and knees, over six weeks.

99 Soft-tissue swellings of both wrists in a 10-year-old, which are tending to sublux.

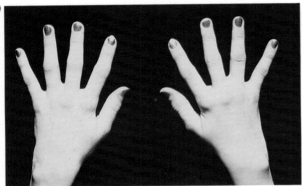

100 A 13-year-old presenting with pain and swelling in the wrists and hands. Note the swelling over the ulnar styloid process and involvement of the metacarpophalangeal joints; this developed over 3–4 months.

101 An 11-year-old with marked swelling over the ulnar styloid and carpus, and early swelling over the metacarpophalangeal and proximal interphalangeal joints, causing flexion at the proximal interphalangeal joints.

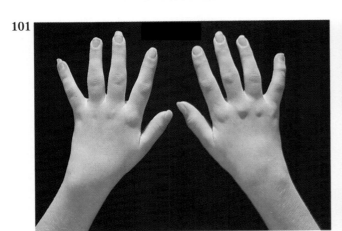

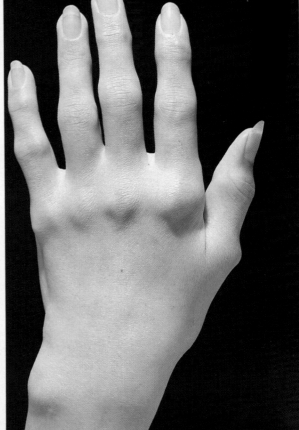

102 A 14-year-old girl with soft-tissue swelling and pain in both wrists, who had undergone a rapid development of metacarpophalangeal joint subluxation in the preceding 6 months.

103 This 13-year-old had a particularly prolific synovitis affecting wrists, over the ulnar styloid, and all the metacarpo- and proximal interphalangeal joints.

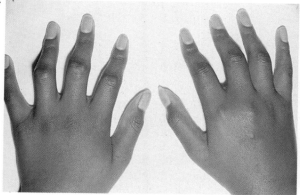

104 Onset of seropositive disease in a West Indian girl, aged 10; note the very marked swelling and flexion of the proximal interphalangeal joints and swelling over the metacarpophalangeal joints.

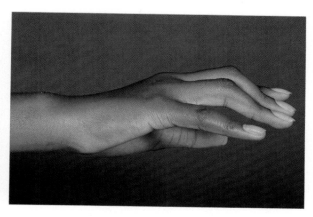

105 Lateral view of **104**, showing inability to dorsiflex the wrist and marked flexion deformity of the proximal interphalangeal joints.

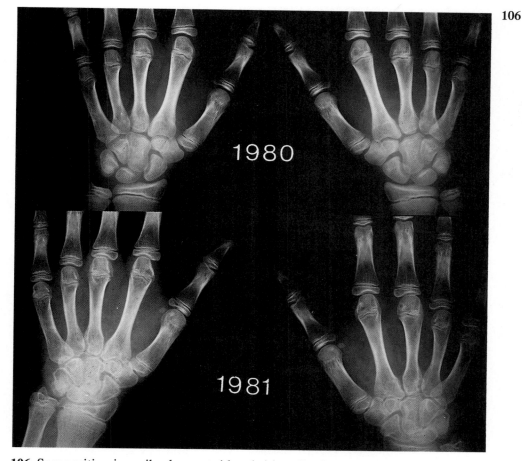

106 Seropositive juvenile rheumatoid arthritis, affecting the wrist predominantly. By 6 months of the illness, crowding of the carpus is obvious, particularly on the left, and there is narrowing of the carpo–metacarpal joint space. After 1 year, there has been very marked deterioration in the state of the carpal bones, with commencing fusion onto the metacarpals and narrowing of metacarpophalangeal joints 2 and 3 bilaterally.

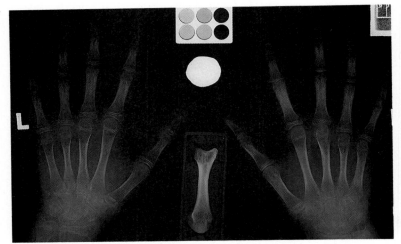

107 Hand X-ray just under 12 months from onset of the first symptom; note dissolution of the carpii, with erosions crowding and overlap onto the metacarpals. The second metacarpophalangeal joint also shows slight radial deviation. The third metacarpophalangeal joints, right and left, show a narrowing of the joint space and early erosion.

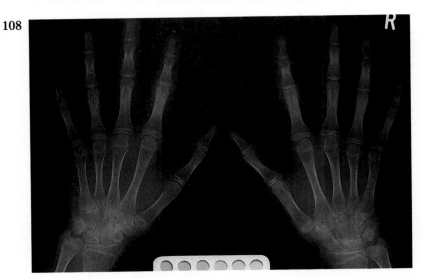

108 The same patient as in **107**, 1 year later, after gold therapy. There is some improvement in the carpal state, but more widespread erosions have occurred at the metacarpophalangeal level.

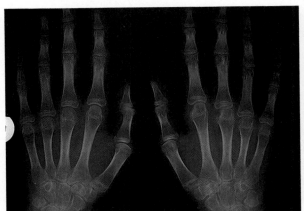

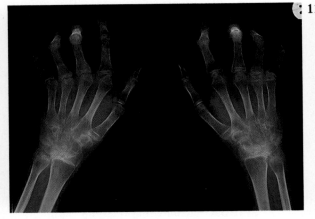

109, 110 An X-ray (**109**) of an 11-year-old taken 1 year from the first symptom, showing extensive erosions, with narrowing of joint spaces at the metacarpophalangeal joints; there is severe osteoporosis around these joints, and the proximal interphalangeal joints have become narrowed. **110** is an X-ray of the same patient 1 year later. There has been considerable further destruction, despite intramuscular gold.

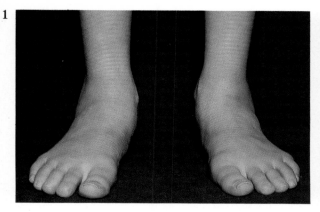

111 Soft-tissue swelling of the ankles. Early valgus deformity of the hind feet and soft-tissue swelling across the metatarsophalangeal joints, all of which developed in the preceding 6 months, making walking extremely painful.

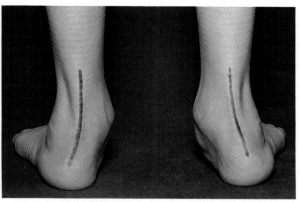

112 Back view of the case in **111** showing the severity of the valgus deformity.

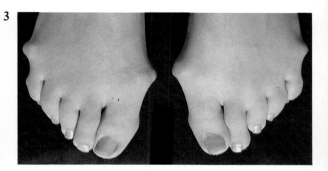

113 Soft-tissue swelling of metatarsophalangeal joints with nodule formation over the bony prominences of the first and fifth metatarsophalangeal joints.

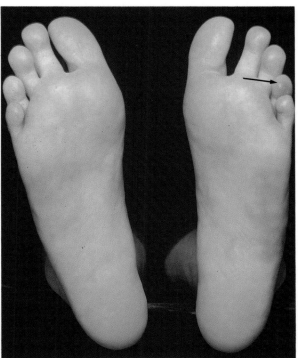

114 This girl, whose illness commenced at 9 years of age, exhibits a marked difference in size of her two feet; note also the mottling of the soles of the feet and vasculitic lesions in the toe pads (arrow).

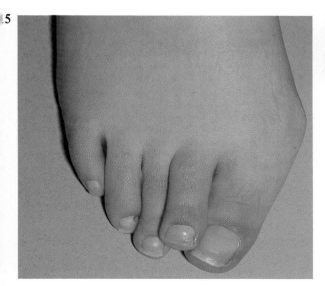

115 This Indian girl was 8 years old at the onset of symptoms, and rapidly developed a growth defect in the second toe and marked hallux valgus at the first metatarsophalangeal joint.

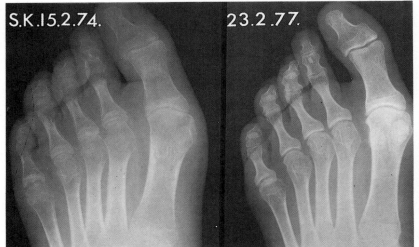

116 Marked osteoporosis around the metatarsophalangeal joints, with erosions in the fifth, and crowding of the joint space (left X-ray). After treatment with penicillinamine there was a remarkable improvement in this 13-year-old girl's state, and by 3 years (right X-ray) there had been healing of the erosions in the feet, and the restoration of a more normal function, although a slight hallux valgus persisted.

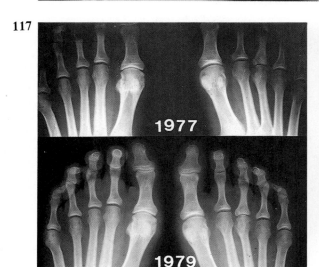

117 Erosion in metatarsophalangeal joints (left X-ray) at presentation 6 weeks after the first complaint of pain in a 13-year-old girl who was strongly rheumatoid factor positive. Started on chloroquine, with benefit and healing of the erosion over 2 years (right X-ray).

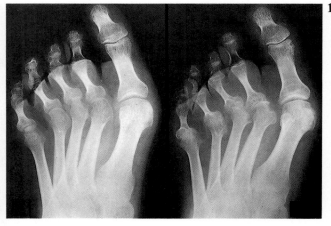

118 Despite intramuscular gold, there was progressive radiological change over 5 years in this 15-year-old girl's feet.

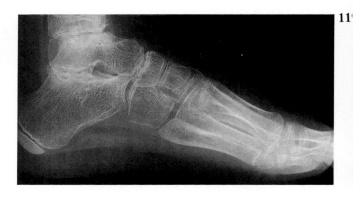

119 Erosive change in the ankle joint, partial collapse of the talus, and narrowing with erosions in talo–navicular and talo–calcaneal joints.

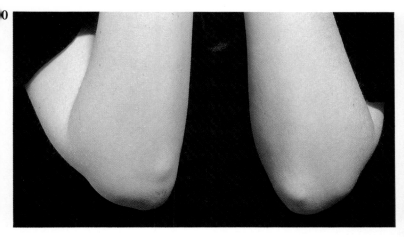

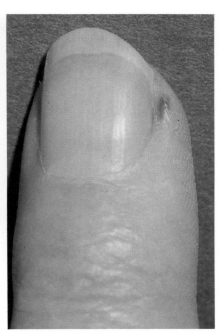

120 Nodules on the elbows. Note that one is on the point of the elbow and the other further down the forearm. Histologically, these look like those of adult rheumatoid arthritis.

121 Typical nail fold lesions.

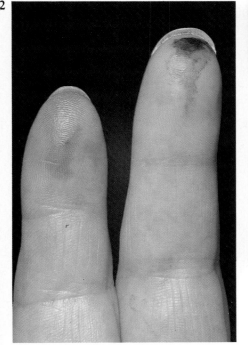

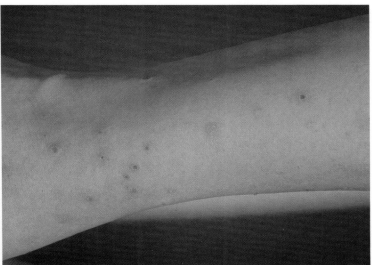

123 Vasculitic rash along the arm in Jamaican girl.

122 Vasculitic lesions in the pads of the fingers.

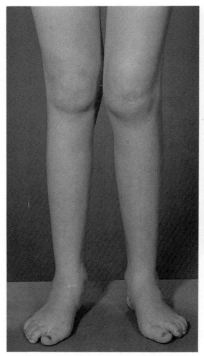

124 A 13-year-old with knee problems of 1 year's duration.

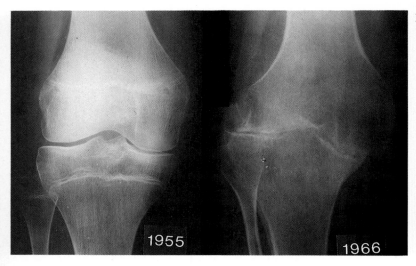

1955   1966

125 Overgrowth of the medial femoral condyle with narrowing of the joint space 1 year from onset in a 14-year-old. Despite long-acting drugs, progressive destruction occurred over 11 years.

126 A 7-year-old with swelling of the right knee, followed over a few months by the left. In the top X-ray, 1 year from onset both knees show narrowing of the joint space, alteration in the growth of the femoral epiphyses, with overgrowth of the medial femoral condyle, and erosions. This proceeded over the next 2 years, with the right leg being more severely affected than the left by overgrowth, flexion contracture and further radiological deterioration.

127 A teenager suffering from juvenile rheumatoid arthritis of 18 months' duration, showing ossification within the synovial membrane in the suprapatellar pouch. No corticosteroid injections had been given.

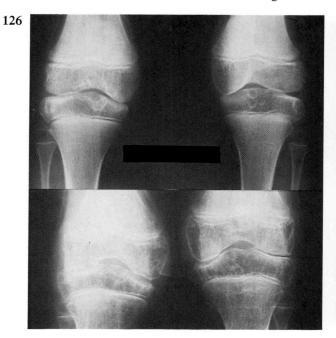

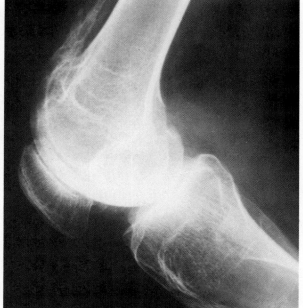

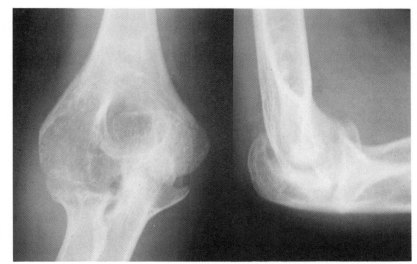

128 This elbow X-ray from a girl with onset when 11 years old shows overgrowth of the radial head together with narrowing of the joint space and marked erosion, 3 years after her first symptoms. She now re-presented with ulnar nerve symptoms of numbness and tingling in the fifth finger from pressure on the ulnar nerve.

129 Serious hip destruction over 3 years in a 13-year-old boy.

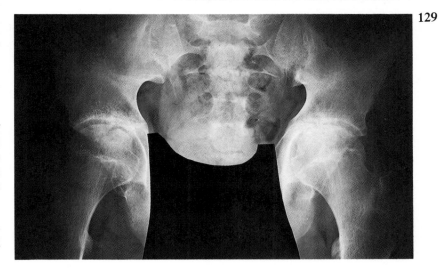

130 After 5 years from onset of her disease, this now 13-year-old girl woke one morning unable to stand, and she complained that her legs would not hold her; note the AA subluxation.

131 Rupture of the extensor tendons to the second and third fingers.

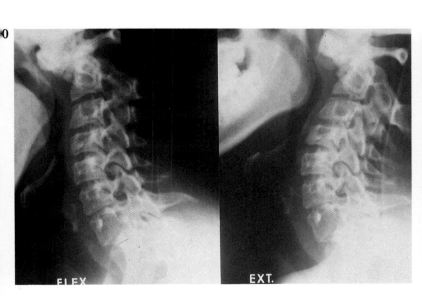

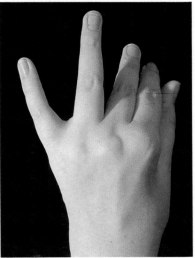

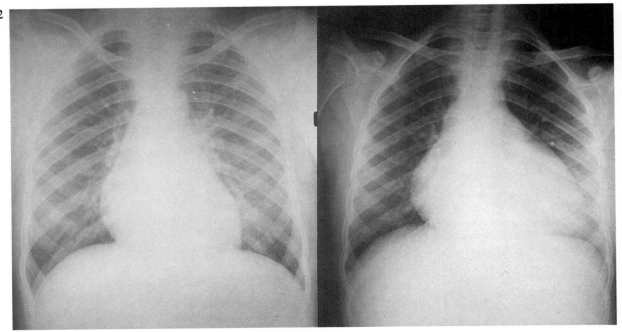

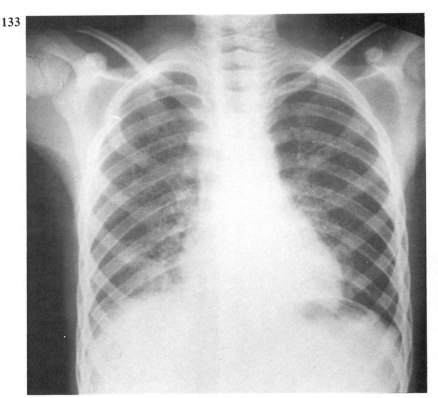

132 This 14-year-old had suffered seropositive juvenile rheumatoid arthritis for 4 years and had been found to have a systolic murmur some 3 months earlier, followed by the development of an early aortic diastolic murmur some 3 months before the left X-ray was taken. Over the next 3 months her cardiac condition rapidly deteriorated, with an enlarging left ventricle and a widened pulse pressure (right X-ray). Successful homograft surgery was undertaken on her aorta.

133 This boy presented with dyspnoea on exertion, and commented that he had felt pain in his hands and feet for 2 years. There were minor soft-tissue swellings and early erosions of metacarpo- and metatarsophalangeal joints, together with finger clubbing. Investigation showed restrictive lung disease.

Pauci-Articular Onset: Younger

General characteristics:
- Under 6 years of age
- Girls more than boys

Clinical features:
- Arthritis affecting four or fewer joints: commonly knee, ankle, elbow or a single finger
- Early local growth anomalies
- Risk (1 in 3) of chronic iridocyclitis in the first 5 years of disease

Investigations:
- ESR – may be elevated or normal, initially
- Haemoglobin – normal
- White blood count – normal
- Platelets – normal
- IgM rheumatoid factor – negative
- ANA – frequently positive
- HLA A2, DR5, DRw6, and DRw8

Course and prognosis:
- Exacerbations and remissions
- Alteration in growth of affected limb
- Long-term prognosis of joints good, except for the one in five who develop polyarthritis (nine or more joints) over a period of years
- Iridocyclitis is bilateral in two-thirds, the course is independent of the joints; its prognosis depends on early detection and good management

Management:
- Appropriate splinting
- Physiotherapy to maintain muscle and joint function
- NSAIDs
- Occasional local corticosteroid injection
- Frequent ophthalmological assessment (3–6 monthly)

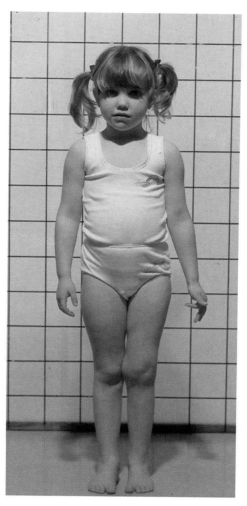

134

134 A 5-year-old who developed acute swelling of the left knee, followed rapidly by some swelling of the right knee and the left ankle. Note the early flexion contracture developing on the left side.

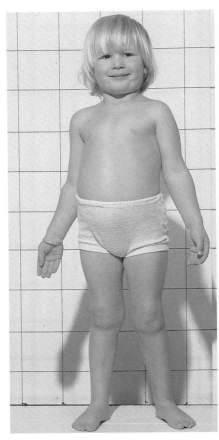

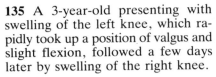

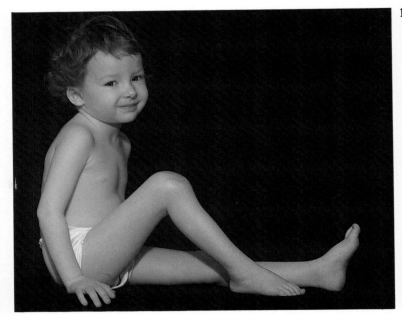

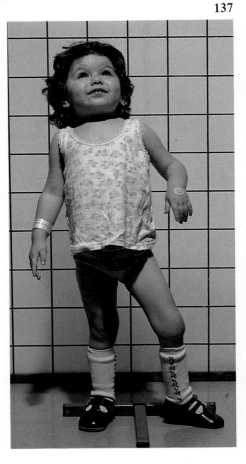

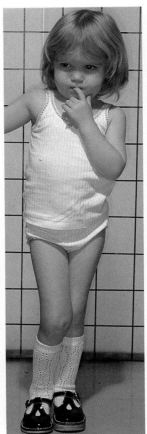

135 A 3-year-old presenting with swelling of the left knee, which rapidly took up a position of valgus and slight flexion, followed a few days later by swelling of the right knee.

136 A 3-year-old presenting with acute swelling of the right knee and refusal to extend the knee.

137 A 3-year-old presenting with rapidly developing flexion deformity of the left knee, associated with valgus deformity of the left ankle. The left knee is held in a position of external rotation at the hip, with flexion and valgus occurring at the knee.

138 A 3-year-old presenting with pain, swelling and flexion deformity of the right knee.

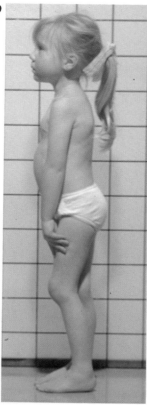
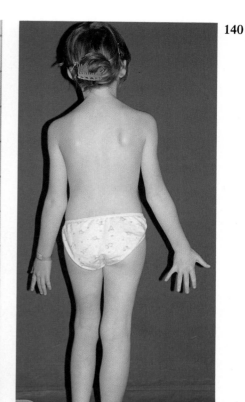

139 A 4-year-old presenting with swelling and inability to extend the left knee.

140 Persistent flexion contracture of the left knee. Note the marked wasting of leg and early scoliosis.

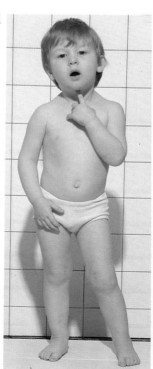
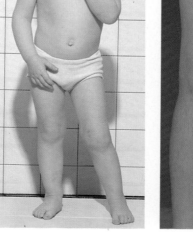
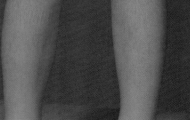

141 A 3-year-old boy with a 2-week history of swelling of the left knee and difficulty in using the limb; note the flexion and valgus deformity.

142 A close-up of monarticular arthritis, showing severe soft-tissue swelling and a large effusion with commencing overgrowth of the femur.

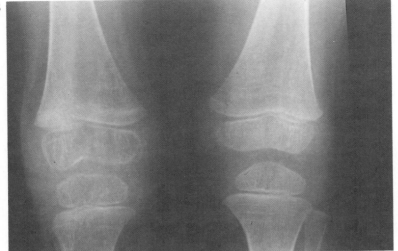

143 X-ray of the patient in **136**, showing alteration in the growth of the epiphysis and, to a lesser extent, the metaphysis 6 months after the first symptom: flexion deformity exaggerates the apparent size of the epiphyses. There was already a 1 cm difference in leg length.

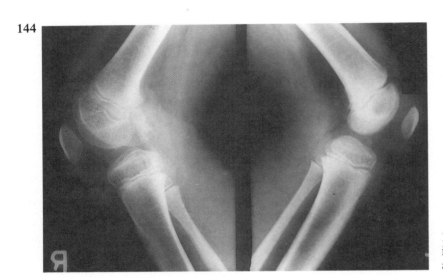

144 Lateral X-ray of knees, showing overgrowth of the patella on the affected side 6 months from onset.

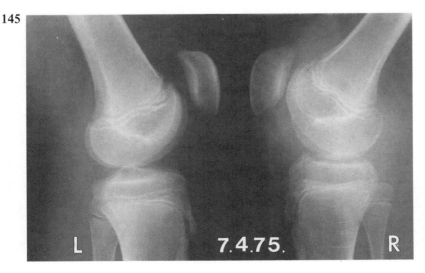

145 Marked overgrowth of the patella and femoral epiphysis, which occurred over 3 years. The other knee had been affected for 9 months, with commencing change in the patella.

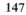

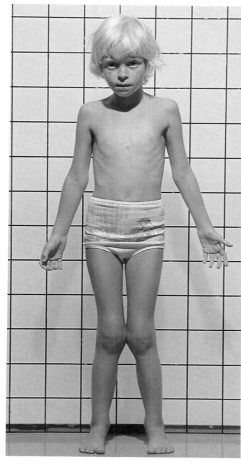

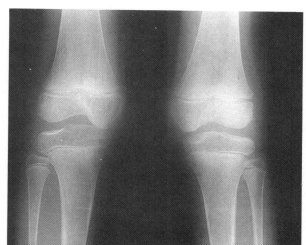

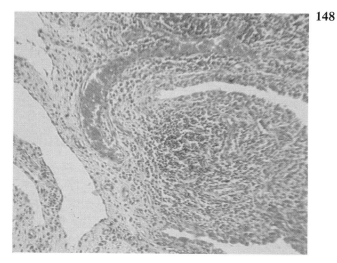

146 This 6-year-old girl presented with pain and swelling in the right knee, followed a few months later by the same in the left knee. Note the early flexion and contractures and slight valgus deformity.

147 X-ray of the child shown in **146**, showing overgrowth, especially of the medial femoral condyle, and widening of the condylar notch, particularly marked on the first-affected side (right). This is 1 year from onset.

148 Histology of the synovial membrane in a girl with a single swollen knee, showing marked hyperplasia and inflammatory cell infiltration, predominantly mononuclear (*haematoxylin and eosin, H & E*).

149 Acute deformity of the ankle in a young child, commencing some 6 weeks previously; she refused to stand on her leg.

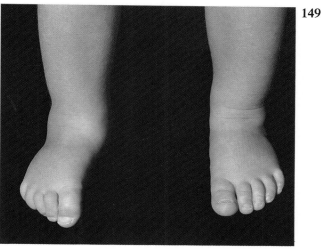

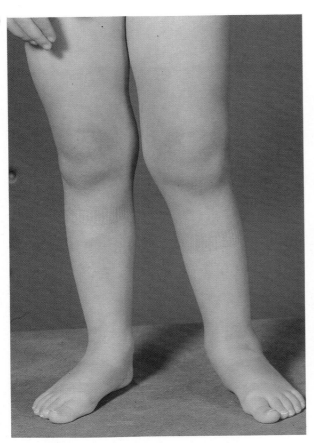

150 A close-up of a leg of a 3-year-old who started with pain and swelling in the left ankle, followed by the same in the left knee. Note that both the knee and ankle have taken up a valgus position.

151 Bone scan of a child with the left ankle and hind foot showing a marked increase in uptake in both sites compared with the normal right ankle.

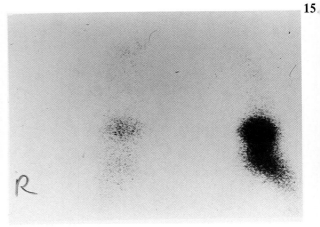

R

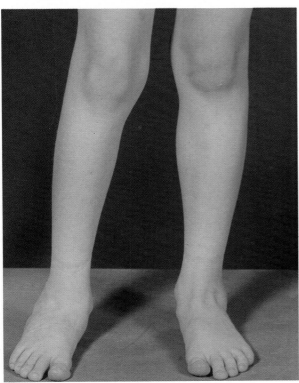

152 Presentation of a 4-year-old boy with pain, swelling and the rapid development of deformity of the right foot; note the valgus position.

153 Close-up of **152** showing the soft-tissue swelling extending over the ankle onto the foot.

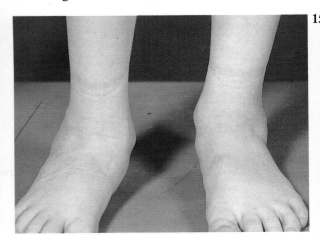

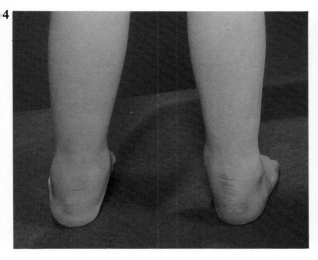

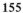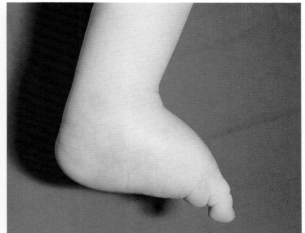

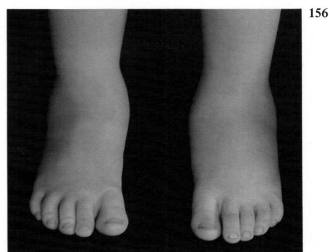

154 A 2-year-old presenting with swelling of the right ankle, which is already taking up a valgus position. This was followed by swelling of the left ankle.

155 Acute swelling of the whole foot in an 8-month-old boy who disliked any pressure on the foot.

156 This 3-year-old had bilateral severe ankle swelling following presentation with a single knee two weeks previously.

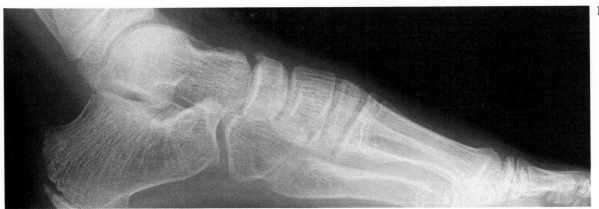

157 Lateral foot X-ray 6 years after pauci-articular onset involving ankle and hind foot. Disease now quiescent. Note reasonable bone texture but narrowing of talo-navicular joint with a bony spur forming.

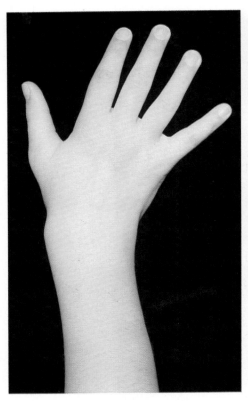

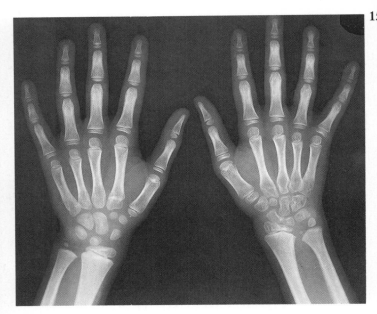

159 X-ray of patient in **158**. There is slight change in the development of the ulna, osteoporosis and slight overgrowth of the carpus on the affected side. Note the impaired growth of the whole hand.

158 Unilateral wrist involvement is associated with ulna deviation at wrist level, presumably due to muscle spasm as it precedes any overt growth defect.

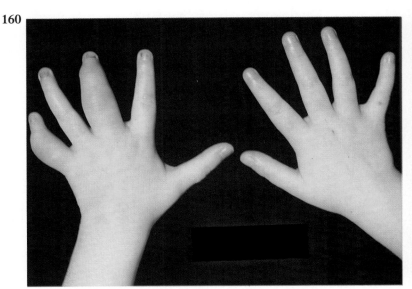

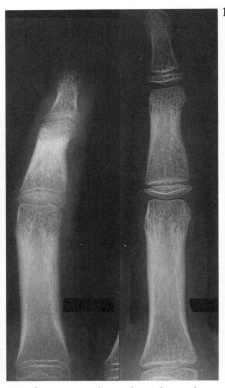

160 Severe flexor tenosynovitis with slight swelling of joints, particularly affecting the third and fifth fingers on the right hand. Note the early flexion deformity.

161 Osteoporosis and periosteal reaction in an older girl at the site of flexor tenosynovitis (left); note the regression after 1 year (right).

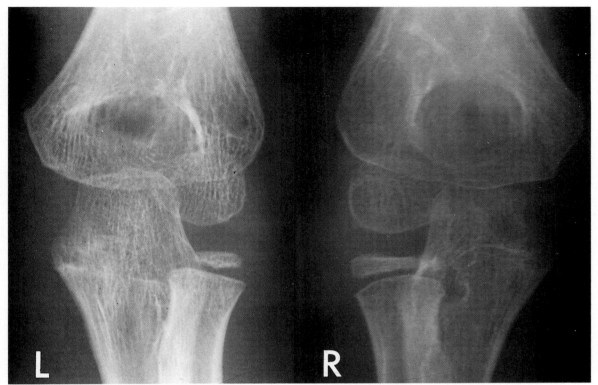

162 The elbow as a presenting site: 8 months after swelling and limitation was first noted, osteoporosis and changes in growth have occurred, particularly an increase in the radial epiphysis of the affected right elbow.

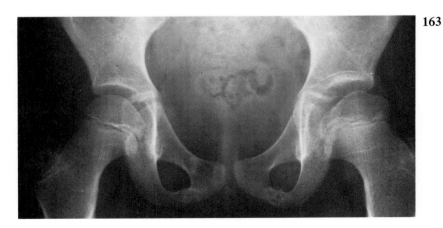

163 Rarely, unilateral hip involvement causes alteration in the growth of the femoral head with coxa magna, and widening and shortening of the femoral neck.

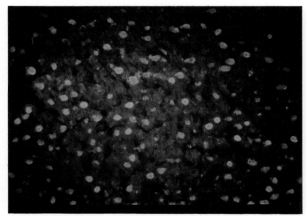

164 Positive ANA test on rat liver.

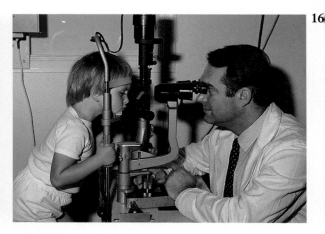

165 Slit-lamp examination of the eye by Mr J. Kanski, FRCS; this is mandatory in all young onset pauci-articular disease and needs to be repeated every 2–3 months if the ANA test is positive.

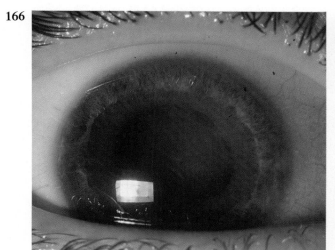

166 Eye containing pigmentary deposits and the commencement of cataract.

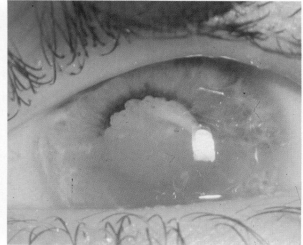

167 Typical triad of chronic iridocyclitis, band opacity, pigmentary deposits due to previous inflammation, and cataract.

Pauci-Articular Onset: Older (Juvenile Spondyloarthropathy)

General characteristics:
- 9 years old and over
- Male predominance

Clinical features:
- Peripheral arthritis predominantly affecting the joints of the lower limbs
- Enthesopathies – plantar fascia, Achilles tendon, patella tendon
- Acute iritis
- Sacroiliac pain in some ⎫ Either of these can be
- Axial disease in some ⎭ the presenting feature

Investigations:
- ESR – normal to high
- Full blood count – usually normal
- IgM rheumatoid factor – negative
- HLA B27 – present

Course and prognosis:
- Functional outcome good in two-thirds of cases
- Some joint extension may occur
- Over time a third can develop serious hip problems, cervical and other spinal involvement, impaired temporomandibular function, as well as other features of spondylitis

Management:
- Physiotherapy, including hydrotherapy, to maintain mobility: particularly important if spinal involvement occurs
- Posture training
- NSAIDs
- Local corticosteroid injections
- Hip arthroplasty may be needed in a small proportion

168

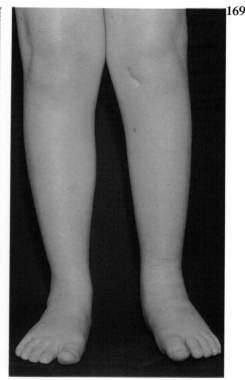

169

168 A boy of 12 presenting with bilateral knee effusions and slight swelling of the left ankle, which had been present for 4 months. His mother had suffered acute iridocyclitis; the boy carried HLA B27.

169 This 11-year-old boy presented with what was thought to be a 'spastic' left foot. He was put into plaster, but when the plaster was removed some 6 weeks later he had a persistent valgus deformity of the foot, which had become immobile; note the severe wasting of the calf.

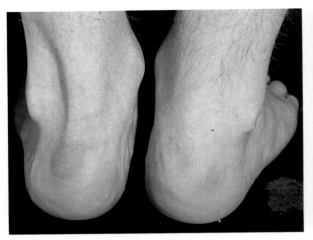

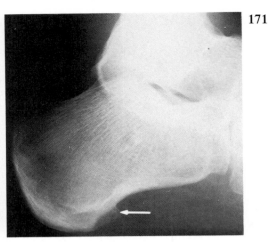

170 This 13-year-old boy presented with persistent pain in the heel and difficulty in walking. Clinically, he had thickening round the tendo Achilles and marked tenderness of the plantar fascia.

171 A large spur (arrow) developing as a result of plantar fascia fasciitis.

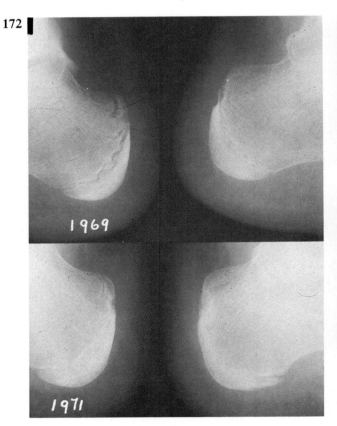

1969

1971

172 Development of erosive lesions at the os calcis as a sequel to tendo Achilles involvement.

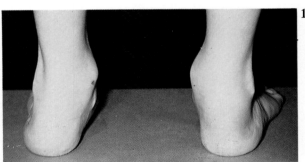

173 This 12-year-old presented with pain in both heels and ankles, and difficulty in walking; note the valgus deformity and the thickening of the tendo Achilles.

174 This 13-year-old boy had already had an attack of irritable hip, first on the right and then on the left side, which had recovered. He now re-presented with pain in the ankle, and was found to have a tendon sheath effusion along the medial malleolus.

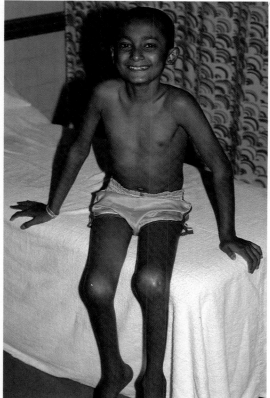

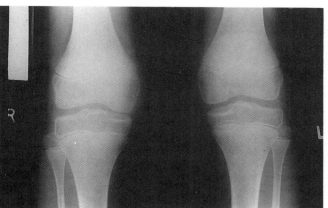

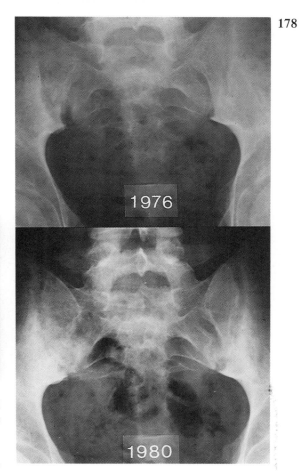

175 This 11-year-old Indian boy presented with bilateral knee swelling and effusions, and ankle involvement. He had rapidly developed knee contractures over 6 months.

176 Overgrowth of the epiphyses of the right affected knee in an adolescent with unilateral involvement of 18 months' duration.

177 Progressive bony changes as a sequel to enthesopathies, affecting the tibial tubercle and the inferior and superior poles of the patella in a boy with probable juvenile spondylitis.

178 Initially, the sacroiliac joints are usually normal, but over a 4–5-year period, as shown here, there is a gradual development of sacro-iliitis.

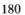

179

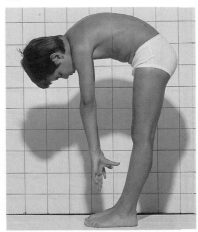

180

181

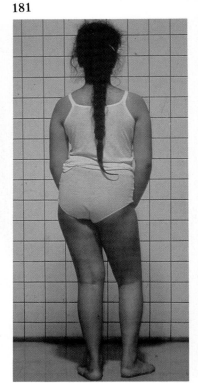

179 This 10-year-old boy presented with pain and slight swelling of the left ankle.

180 The same boy as in **179** had normal back movement.

181 Although hip presentation is more common in older boys, it can also occur in girls, causing difficulty in walking and sometimes a flexion contracture.

182

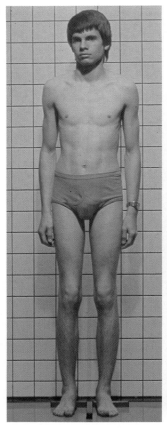

183

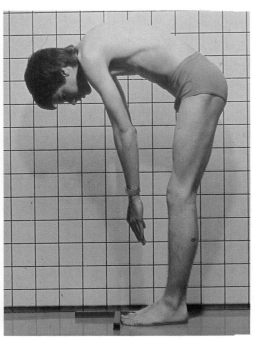

182 This 14-year-old boy presented with pain and difficulty in extending both knees and elbows. His father suffered from ankylosing spondylitis.

183 The patient in **182** had no complaint of back pain, but note limitation of the thoracolumbar spine, indicating that he, too, has ankylosing spondylitis.

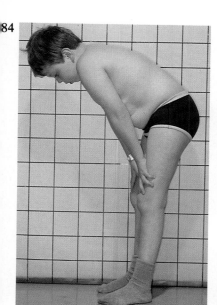

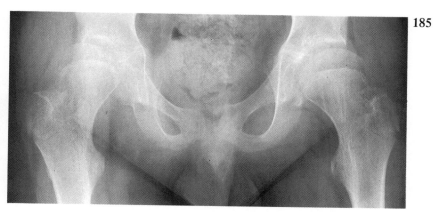

184 Note the difficulty in flexing the hips, but normal rounding of the back.

185 Bilateral enlargement of the femoral heads of the patient in **184**, with a tendency to lateral subluxation. This boy had suffered an onset of recurrent hip pain 2 years earlier when 8 years old. The age of onset modifies, to some extent, the pattern of radiological change.

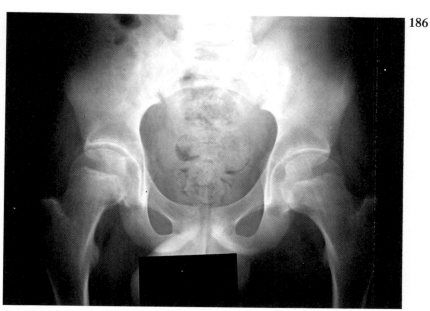

186 This boy, aged 11 years, had an onset with hip pain; note the tendency to enlargement of the femoral heads, together with joint space narrowing.

187 This 14-year-old boy presented with pain and loss of movement of the left hip, of 9 months' duration; note the normally shaped acetabulae, the change in shape of the femoral heads on both sides, and particularly the apparent slight elongation of the left femoral head.

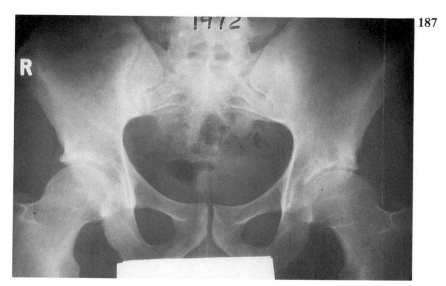

59

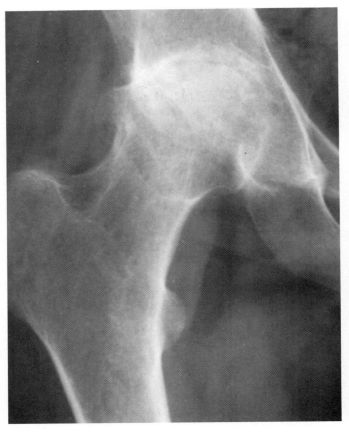

188 The hip shown in this X-ray belongs to a girl who had an onset with neck pain at the age of 11. Here, at 15, she has progressive problems in the hip, which shows marked loss of joint space. Note the overall enlargement and elongation of the femoral head and the ruff-like state around the femoral neck.

189 Loss of movement in both spine and hip joints in an Indian boy who had presented with knee effusions 5 years previously, when 10 years old.

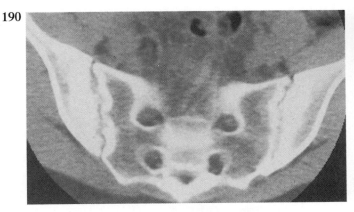

190 A CAT scan showing irregularity of sacroiliac joints in a patient who showed minimal radiological changes.

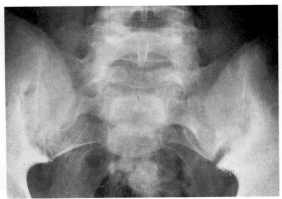

191 Sclerosis of sacroiliac joints in a routine X-ray.

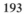

193

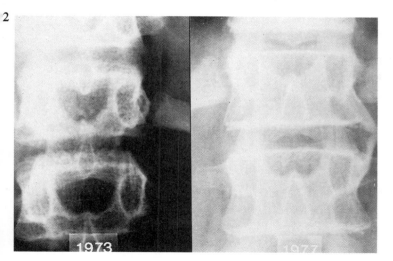

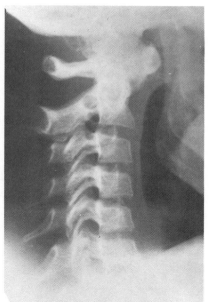

4

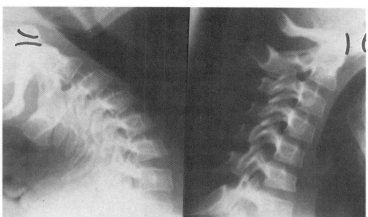

195

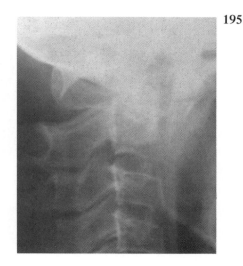

192 Spinal X-ray showing early syndesmophyte formation, which has developed over a 4-year period; note that ring epiphyses are still present, which shows that the patient is still in the adolescent age group.

193 This 8-year-old boy presented with acute pain in the neck and difficulty in lifting his head. In the preceding 6 weeks he had suffered intermittent swelling of the left knee. His father suffered from ankylosing spondylitis. Atlantoaxial subluxation is shown here.

194 The extent of the mobility of the subluxation is shown in these flexion (left) and extension (right) X-rays of the same patient as in **193**.

195,196 This Indian boy, 13 years old, presented with pain in the neck and a torticollis. The torticollis impedes the X-ray view (**195**) of the atlantoaxial joint. Tomography (**196**) confirmed the atlantoaxial subluxation; note the early changes in the sacroiliac joints.

196

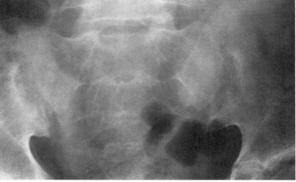

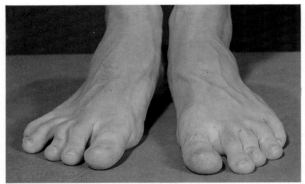

197 After presentation with pain in the ankles and early valgus deformity, this patient complained of pain in the toes; note the clawing of all the toes.

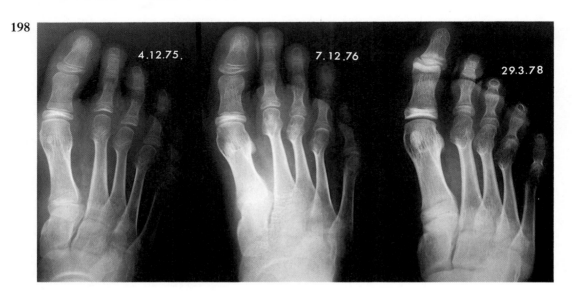

4.12.75.   7.12.76   29.3.78

198 Progressive subluxation without serious erosive disease.

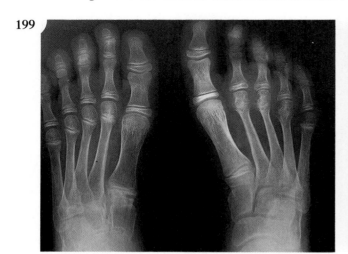

199 Marked erosive changes in left metatarsal heads, particularly 3 and 4.

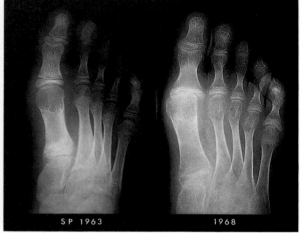

SP 1963   1968

200 Shown here are the changes, over a 5-year period, mainly in the great toe and, to a lesser extent, in the metatarsophalangeal joints. Note the dumb-bell appearance of the metatarsal heads.

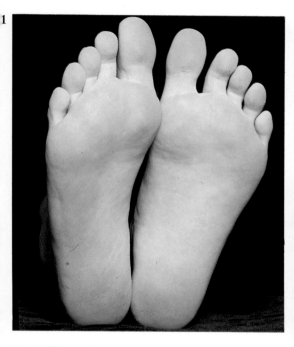

201 Differential foot growth due to unilateral involvement.

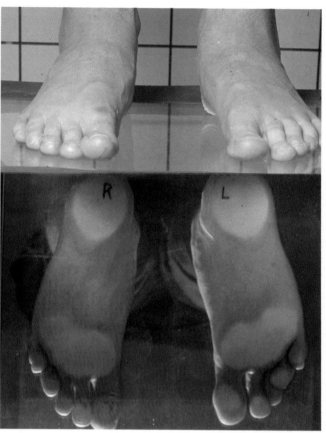

202 This 14-year-old had previously had an episode of so-called irritable hip, which lasted for 4 months, followed by an effusion in the right knee. He then presented with pain in both feet. Note that he has not adopted the normal stance, with most of the foot pressure on the heel and some on the metatarsal heads; this was due to mid-tarsal involvement.

203 This 9-year-old boy presented with pain and rapid deformity in the feet; note the valgus deformity of the hind foot and the flexion deformity of the first metatarsophalangeal joint.

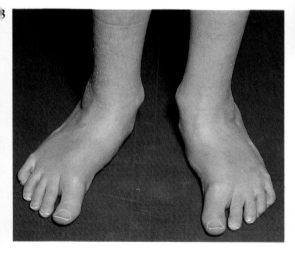

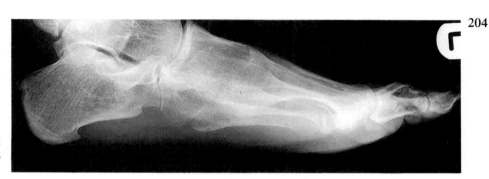

204 Fusion of the distal tarsal bones to the bases of the metatarsal bones.

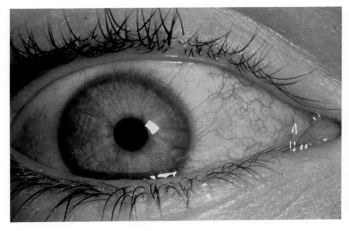

205 The course of the disease is frequently punctuated by attacks of acute iridocyclitis.

206 RAHA negative   Male   Date of birth: 4 May 1958
ANA negative
HLA B27 present
ESR   47   79   64   54   10   5   2

Minor limitation
thoracolumbar spine

Sacroiliitis

Acute iritis   Right

Left subtalar and pain limitation

Left ankle STS

Left knee STS flexed

July 1971   1972   1976   1986

206 The course of this disease in a patient presenting as a peripheral arthropathy, which recovered only to be followed by the later development of ankylosing spondylitis (STS, soft tissue swelling).

207 Male   Date of birth: 1 August 1955

Neck limitation

Temporomandibular pain and limitation

Heel pain

Limitation of thoracic and lumbar spine

Bilateral arthroplasties

Hips

Right knee   Synovectomy

Left knee

Left ankle

1965   1970   1975   1980   1985
Year

207 This boy developed severe hip disease when 12 years old, which was followed by the rapid loss of movement in his spine. This loss occurs in about 15% of cases.

Pauci-Articular Onset Unclassified

Characteristics:
- No association with antinuclear antibodies
- HLA B27 not present
- No iridocyclitis.

- Included within this are a group, predominantly female, aged 6–10 years at onset, with knee involvement, and with a good prognosis.

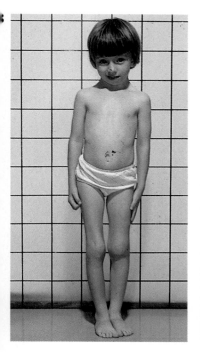

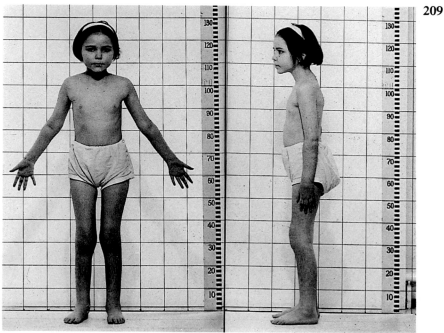

208 This 5½-year-old girl developed swelling of the left knee, which started to flex: 6 weeks later her right knee swelled. The ESR was 9mm/h and ANA proved negative. During a 5-year follow-up no other joints became involved, although activity persisted in the left knee for over 3 years.

209 A 7-year-old who presented with bilateral knee effusion, which caused contracture: the only abnormality was an ESR of 24mm/h. Over the next 5 years complete recovery to straight, fully functional knees occurred, and these have remained so to date (12 years).

JUVENILE PSORIATIC ARTHRITIS

General characteristics:
- An arthritis associated but not necessarily coincident with a typical psoriatic rash, or arthritis, plus at least three of four minor criteria: dactylitis, nail pitting, psoriatic-like rash or family history of psoriasis (Southwood, 1989)
- Female predominance
- Family history of psoriasis (common) or arthritis (but less so)

Clinical features:
- Asymmetrical arthritis
- Flexor tenosynovitis
- Occasionally severe destructive disease
- Systemic features rare
- Nail pitting
- Onycholysis
- Psoriasis

Investigations:
- ESR – varies with number of joints, may be high
- Haemoglobin – may fall
- White blood count – may increase
- IgM rheumatoid factor – negative
- ANA – can be positive

Course and prognosis:
- Young onset can be associated with iridocyclitis
- Remitting and relapsing course, even into adult life
- Occasionally severely destructive
- Occasionally spondylitis develops

Management:
- Physiotherapy
- Splinting as appropriate
- NSAIDs
- Severe destructive form may require immuno-suppressants, such as methotrexate

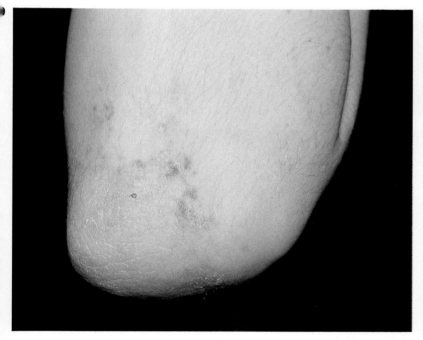

210 Typical patch of psoriasis on the elbow.

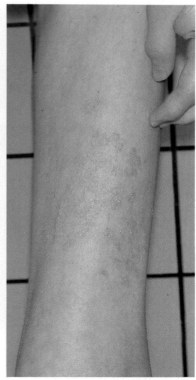

211 Extensive psoriasis along the leg.

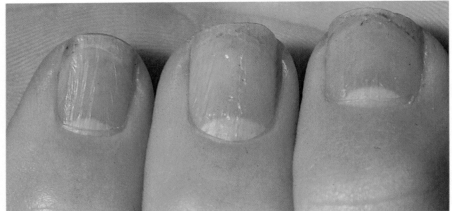

212 Nail pits.

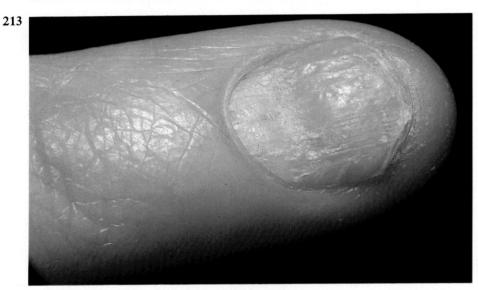

213 Nail pits and some damage to the base of the nail.

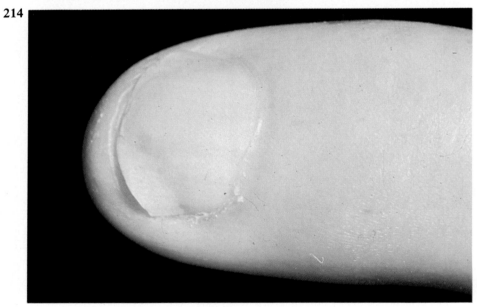

214 Mild subungular atrophy of a finger nail.

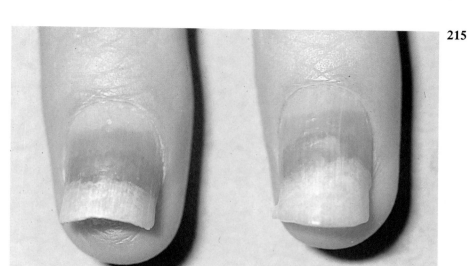

215 Severe subungular atrophy of finger nails.

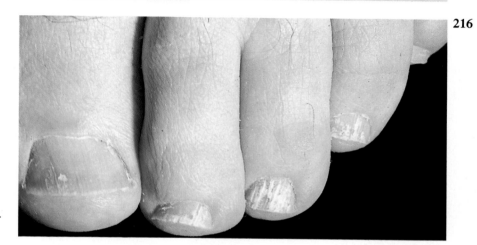

216 Typical subungular atrophy of toenails.

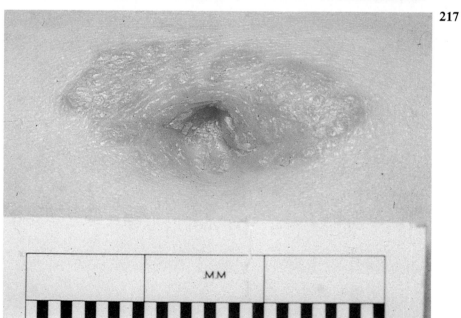

217 Psoriasis around the umbilicus.

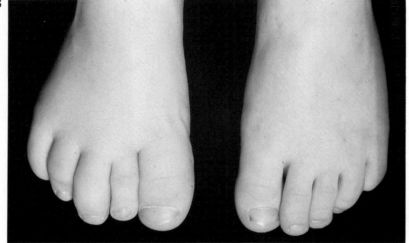

218 A 2½-year-old presenting with overgrowth of the third toe. The toe was painful to touch.

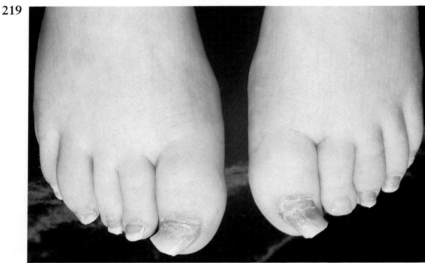

219 Psoriatic arthritis in a boy of 6 years presenting with bilateral swollen great toes associated with nail changes and asymmetrical involvement of other small toe joints.

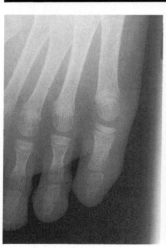
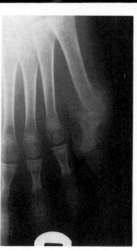

220,221 Periostitis and erosion (**220**) followed by absorption of periostitis and deformity due to joint destruction (**221**) over a 1-year period.

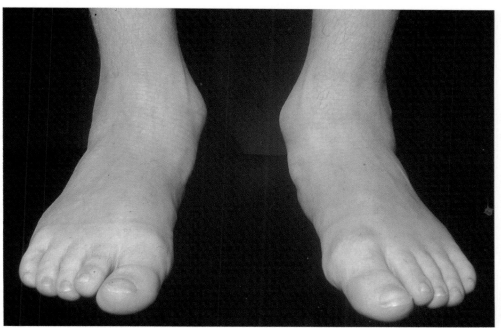

222 Presentation with painful swelling around the ankles associated with tenosynovitis and swelling of first metatarsophalangeal joints of the great toes; note the valgus deformity. The mother suffers from psoriatic arthritis.

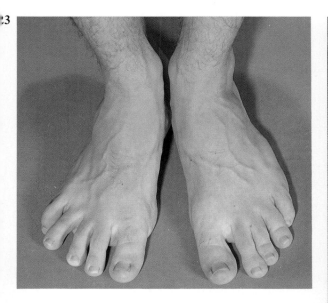

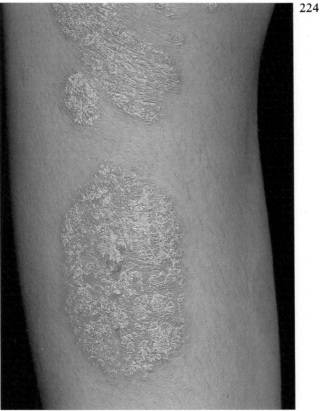

224

223 Adolescent presenting with pain and swelling, particularly of the left ankle, and early valgus deformity; later went on to suffer bilateral sacroiliac changes.

224 Typical scaling psoriatic plaques on the leg.

225

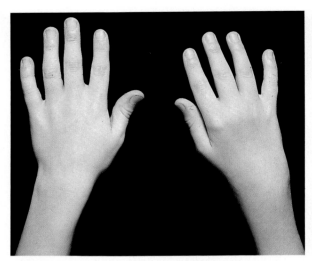

225 Marked asymmetrical involvement with severe changes in the right wrist, swelling and growth defect of the second metacarpophalangeal joint, and swelling of the fourth metacarpophalangeal joint in a 9-year-old boy.

226 X-rays showing predominantly unilateral wrist, carpal and hand involvement, with failure of development of the whole hand.

227 Widespread arthritis. Both knees are involved, but the right is worse than the left; only one wrist, hand and ankle are involved. Note the flexed position of the hip due to bilateral knee involvement.

226

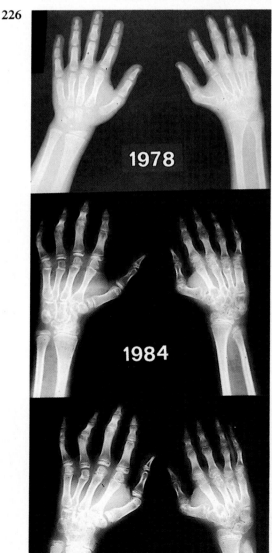

1978

1984

227

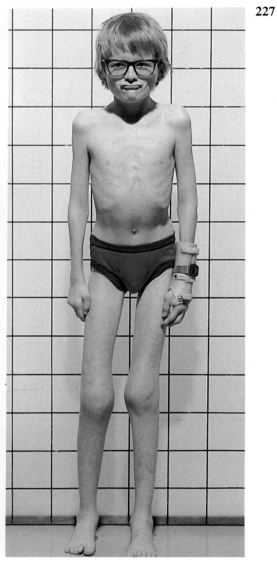

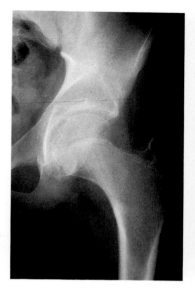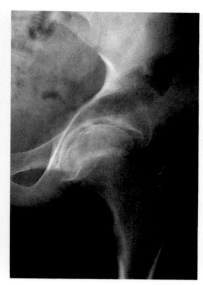

228,229 Onset of psoriasis at age 4. At age 12 there were progressive unilateral hip changes over 3 months. She carried HLA B27.

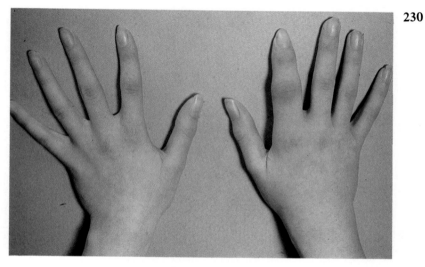

230 Presentation with a single swollen finger in a teenage girl. Note the swelling of the terminal interphalangeal, proximal interphalangeal and metacarpophalangeal joints with tenosynovitis.

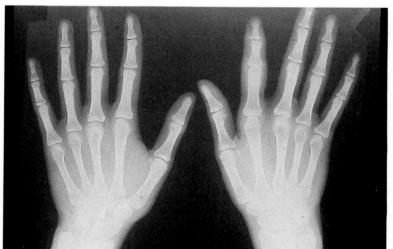

231 X-ray of the hands in **230** showing periosteal reaction and joint space narrowing with erosions in the terminal interphalangeal (TP), proximal interphalangeal and metacarpophalangeal joints of the index finger.

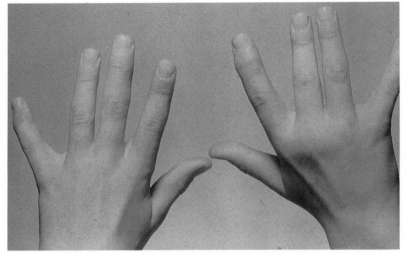

232 A 12-year-old boy presenting with pain and swelling in the hands. Note the asymmetrical involvement with the terminal interphalangeal joint 2, metacarpophalangeal 3, and thumb on the left side and flexor tenosynovitis of the terminal interphalangeal joint of the fifth finger on the right.

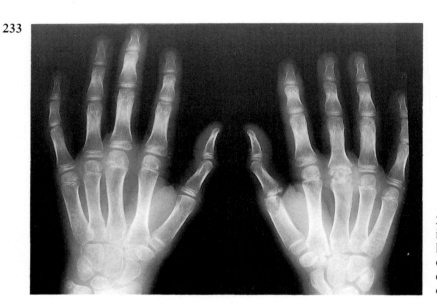

233 X-ray of the case in **232** showing destruction at metacarpophalangeal 3 and loss of alignment and destruction of the thumb metacarpophalangeal joint within 1 year of the first symptoms.

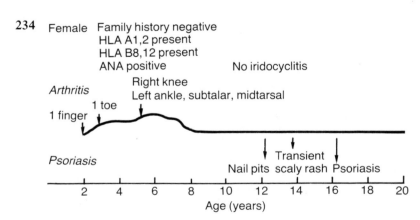

234 Course of disease in a patient, showing the difficulty in diagnosis. There is young onset, with localized and typical joint involvement, followed by gradual recovery and only later the development of psoriasis.

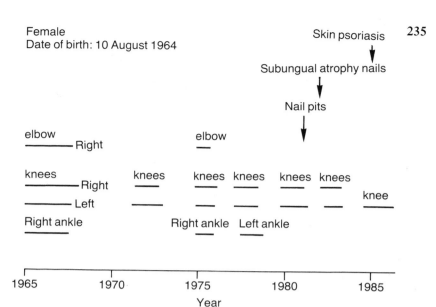

Female
Date of birth: 10 August 1964

Skin psoriasis

Subungual atrophy nails

Nail pits

235 This is a more characteristic course, with recurrent bouts of synovitis, predominantly pauci-articular, with the eventual development of nail changes followed by skin changes. Less than half suffer skin lesions at the onset of joint symptoms.

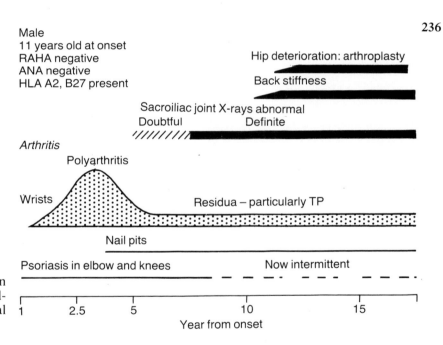

Male
11 years old at onset
RAHA negative
ANA negative
HLA A2, B27 present

236 Course of psoriatic arthritis in an older boy going on to spondylitis (TP, terminal interphalangeal joints).

REACTIVE ARTHRITIS, INCLUDING REITER'S SYNDROME

General characteristics:
- Acute arthritis occurring after an intercurrent infection, without evidence of the causative organism in the joint
- Any age, but particularly teenagers
- Male predominance

Clinical features:
- Arthritis ⎫
- Urethritis/balanitis/cystitis ⎬ Typical triad for Reiter's syndrome
- Conjunctivitis ⎭
- Mouth ulceration
- Fever
- Rashes, including keratodermia blennorrhagica

Investigations:
- ESR – raised
- Haemoglobin – normal
- Mild polymorph leucocytosis
- IgM rheumatoid factor – negative

Investigations (*cont.*):
- ANA – negative
- Occasionally positive stool or urethral culture (*Shigella, Salmonella, Yersinia, Campylobacter, Chlamydia*)
- High incidence of HLA B27

Course and prognosis:
- If only two salient features occur, it is often referred to as 'incomplete Reiter's syndrome'
- Usually self-limiting, but the arthritis can be severe and persistent
- Some may later develop ankylosing spondylitis

Management:
- Antibiotics initially, if an organism is found
- Physiotherapy to maintain function of joints and muscles
- NSAIDs
- Sulphasalazine if joint problems persist

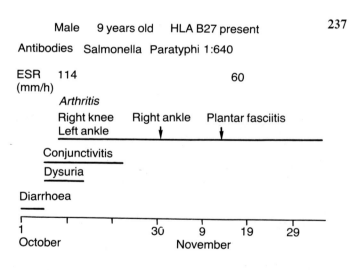

237 Typical course of reactive arthritis

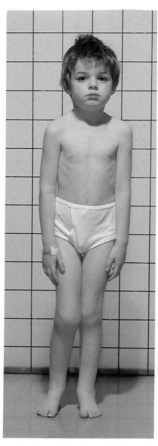

238 Arthritis of the knee and ankle in a young boy who had suffered an episode of diarrhoea and red eye. These were the only clues for a diagnosis of reactive arthritis. He recovered completely within 3 months.

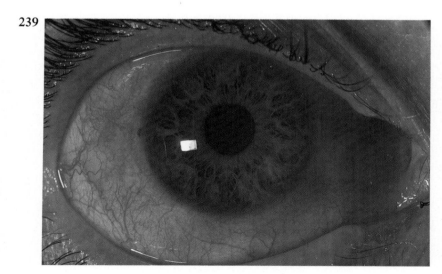

239 Acute conjunctivitis

INFLAMMATORY BOWEL DISEASE

General characteristics:
- Arthritis associated with either ulcerative colitis or Crohn's disease
- Above 4 years of age
- Male and female equal

Clinical features:
- Arthritis usually occurs after the onset of bowel symptoms, but occasionally begins coincident with them, or even precedes them
- Arthritis is usually pauci-articular: knees, ankles, wrists and elbows
- Two forms: (i) benign peripheral arthritis coinciding with active bowel disease; (ii) in older patients who belong to the spondylitic group whose joint activity does not necessarily link with bowel activity

Associated features:
- Erythema nodosum
- Pyoderma gangrenosum
- Mucosal ulcers
- Fever
- Weight loss
- Growth retardation
- Acute iritis – in the spondylitic group

Investigations:
- ESR – usually elevated
- Haemoglobin – usually low
- White blood count – normal
- Platelets – normal
- IgM rheumatoid factor – negative
- ANA – negative
- HLA B27 present in the spondylitic group

Course and prognosis:
- Peripheral arthropathy involves few joints, and is episodic and benign
- Prognosis for joint function is excellent
- Prognosis for the spondylitic group is similar to that of ankylosive spondylitis (p. 58)

Management:
- Physiotherapy as appropriate
- Treatment of the underlying bowel disorder
- NSAIDs with care, because of gastrointestinal side effects (ibuprofen may be the drug of choice)
- Sulphasalazine may be appropriate for both subgroups

240

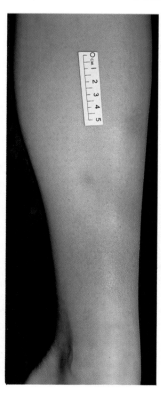

241

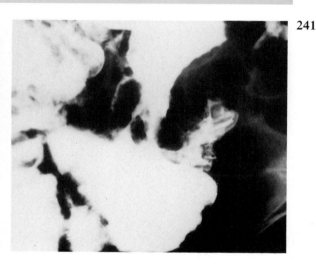

240 Erythema nodosum in a 9-year-old girl who gave a history of general malaise for about 6 weeks, and on examination was found to have not only a raised ESR, but also a haemoglobin level of 10g/l. Further enquiry elicited a description of mild abdominal discomfort with occasionally two or three stools per day. Barium meal and follow-through showed localized regional enteritis.

241 Barium studies showing an area of sclerosis around the region of the appendix.

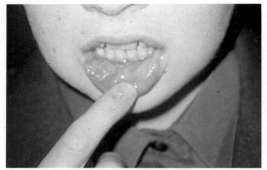

242 Mouth ulcer in a boy who presented with joint pain and minimal swelling of the right knee. The ESR was 64, the haemoglobin 10.8g/l, out of proportion to the degree of synovitis. Mouth ulcers are seen in about 20% of cases of regional enteritis.

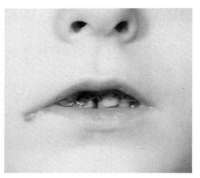

243 Mouth lesions in regional enteritis. (Courtesy of Prof. Walker-Smith, UK.)

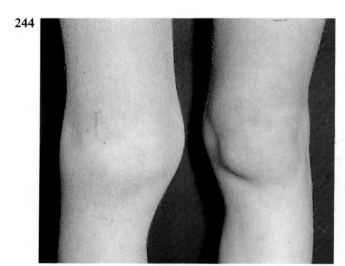

244 Persistent monarticular arthritis of one knee with early flexion deformity. The haemoglobin level fell and ESR rose; abdominal symptoms were minimal, with only occasional bouts of colic; but the patient's stools persistently contained occult blood, and he failed to thrive.

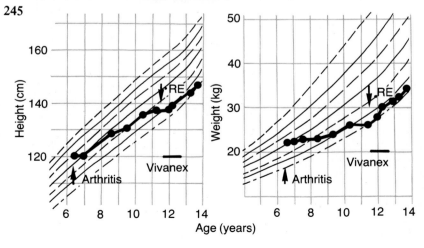

245 An example of failure to gain appropriate weight and height, for which, however, a diagnosis was difficult to establish, despite a barium meal. The diagnosis was finally established by a colonoscopy (RE, regional enteritis).

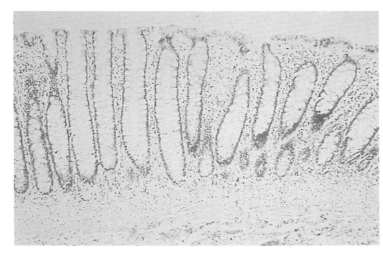

246 Rectal biopsy from a normal subject; note the symmetrical crypts with abundant goblet mucus cells (*H & E, × 100*). (Courtesy of Dr R.J. Grand, USA.)

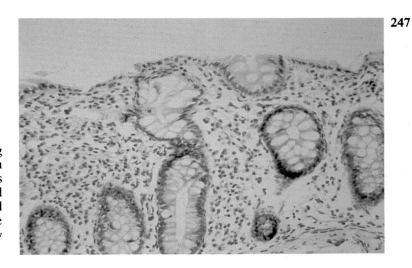

247 Sigmoid biopsy obtained during colonoscopy of a 15-year-old girl with Crohn's disease. The biopsy shows mild, active colitis with acute and chronic inflammatory infiltrate and some destruction of the surface epithelium (*H & E, × 100*). (Courtesy of Dr R.J. Grand, USA.)

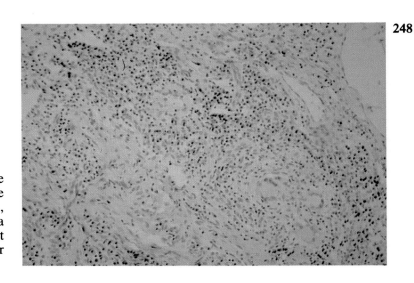

248 Rectal biopsy from the same patient as described in **247**; note the marked destruction of epithelium, acute and chronic inflammation, and a non-caseating granuloma with giant cell (*H & E, × 400*). (Courtesy of Dr R.J. Grand, USA.)

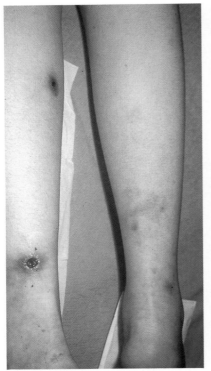
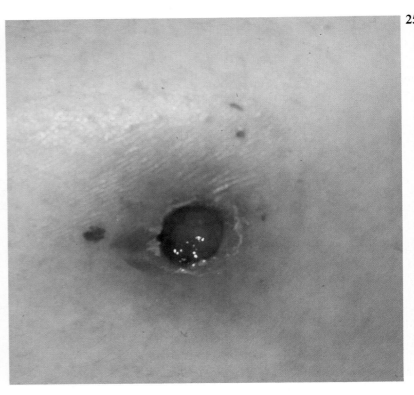

249,250 This 13-year-old girl presented with a mild but widespread polyarthritis, affecting particularly the knees, proximal interphalangeal joints, wrists, elbows and ankles. The ESR was persistently very high, and haemoglobin fell to 8.9g/l. Her stools occasionally contained occult blood. She then developed widespread ulcerating lesions on the lower limbs, **250**, suggestive of pyoderma gangrenosum. Colonoscopy confirmed a diagnosis of regional enteritis in both colon and lower ileum.

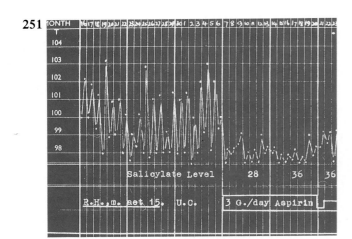

251 Fever chart of a boy who presented with generalized polyarthritis and high fevers, which partly responded to salicylates. There was no rash and no lymphadenopathy or hepatosplenomegaly. His haemoglobin continued to fall, then diarrhoea became obvious, and a barium enema confirmed ulcerative colitis.

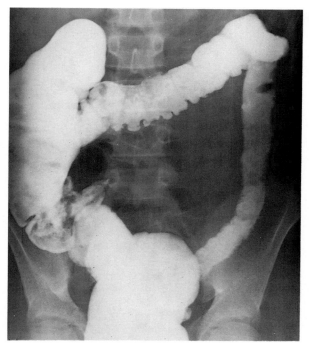

252 Barium enema showing extensive ulcerative colitis in a boy who presented with a peripheral arthropathy and a low-grade fever, but also severe anaemia.

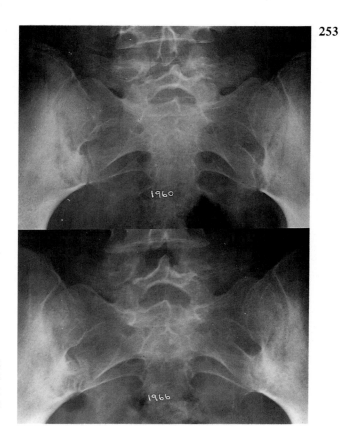

253 Progressive sacroiliac joint changes following presentation as a lower limb arthropathy, with persistent severe anaemia. Despite investigations at regular intervals it took 3 years to diagnose as ulcerative colitis.

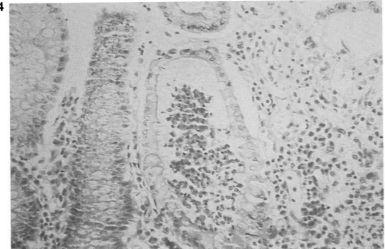

254 Rectal biopsy from an adolescent with ulcerative colitis; note the chronic inflammatory infiltrate in the lamina propria, expanding the intercryptal space (*H & E, × 400*). (Courtesy of Dr R.J. Grand, USA.)

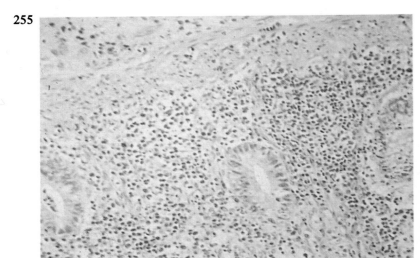

255 Crypt abscess in a rectal biopsy from a 17-year-old with active ulcerative colitis; note the destruction of one crypt and a second distorted crypt with an abundant infiltrate of polymorphonuclear leukocytes; adjacent crypts show depletion of mucus in epithelial cells (*H & E, × 400*). (Courtesy of Dr R.J. Grand, USA.)

RHEUMATIC FEVER

General characteristics:
- An inflammatory reaction in joints, skin, heart and CNS following a Group A haemolytic streptococcal infection
- Age generally over 3 years
- Both sexes, but girls more than boys

Revised Jones' criteria (Stollerman *et al.*, 1965)

Major manifestations	*Minor manifestations*
• Carditis (severe pancarditis can occur in first or subsequent attacks) • Polyarthritis • Erythema marginatum • Subcutaneous nodules • Chorea	• Fever • Arthralgia • Previous rheumatic fever and rheumatic heart disease • Raised acute phase (ESR, C-reactive protein) • Prolonged PR interval on ECG

- Plus supporting evidence of preceding streptococcal infection:
  Throat swab positive for Group A streptococcus, increased antistreptolysin O and anti-DNAase B titres

Investigations:
- ESR – raised if not in cardiac failure
- Haemoglobin – may fall with chronic disease
- White blood count – normal or slight rise
- IgM rheumatoid factor – negative
- ANA – negative
- ECG – may be abnormal
- Echocardiogram – may show valvular or myocardial dysfunction
- Newer scanning techniques may suggest myocarditis

Course and prognosis:
- Average attack lasts 6 weeks
- High risk of recurrence in patients who do not receive adequate prophylaxis against streptococcal infection

Management:
- Bed rest in the acute phase
- Penicillin to eradicate residual streptococcal infection
- Salicylate therapy
- Corticosteroids in patients with significant carditis
- Prophylactic oral or intramuscular penicillin for a minimum of 5 years after an attack, and probably required into adult life.

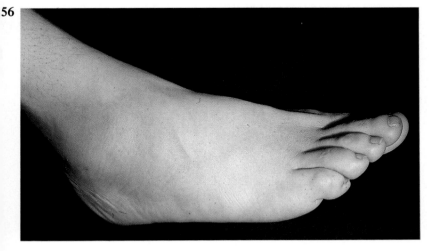

256 Rheumatic fever can present as an arthralgia, mild arthritis, or acutely painful joints, which even mimic septic arthritis. The arthritis is migratory, lasting 2–3 days in one large joint before moving on to another. This shows a red hot, acutely tender ankle in a 10-year-old boy.

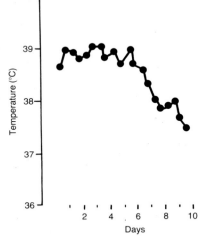

257 A sustained fever that can persist for days, or up to 2–3 weeks, before gradually falling.

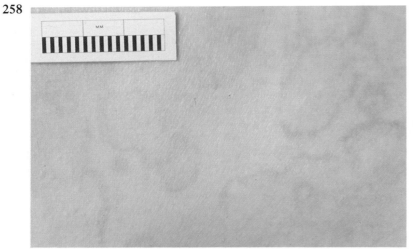

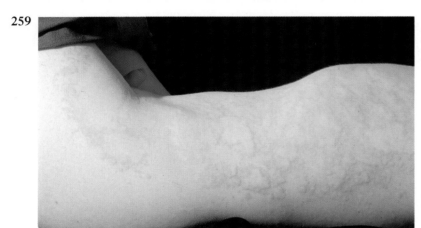

258,259 Typical erythema marginatum. Note the map-like edge of the lesion, which changes from hour to hour.

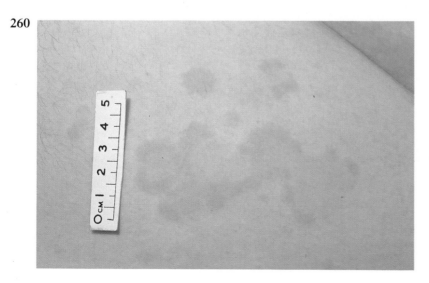

260 Erythema marginatum in which an urticarial element is present.

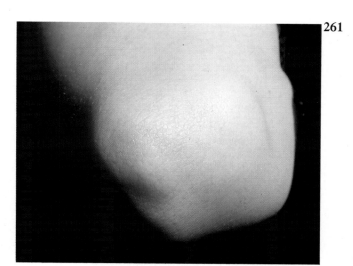

261 A nodule on the elbow. These tend to occur after several weeks of illness. They can develop over any extensor surface and are associated with carditis.

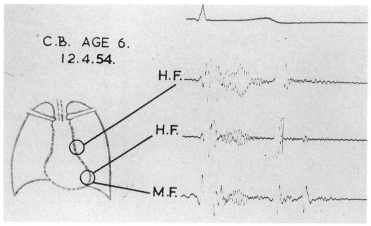

262 A phonocardiograph showing a pansystolic murmur and a soft basal diastolic murmur.

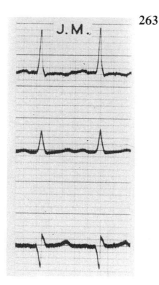

263 ECG of a child with pericarditis, which shows flattening of the T-waves.

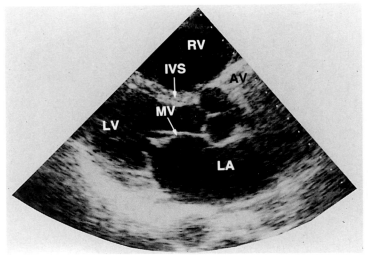

264 This diastolic frame shows a normal aortic valve (closed). The mitral valve (MV), however, is severely thickened, a result of rheumatic fever in childhood. The valve is open, but stenosed and the leaflets have a typical domed appearance. Note the dilatation of the left atrium (IVS, intraventricular septum; RV, right ventricle; LV, left ventricle; AV, aortic valve; LA, left atrium). (Courtesy of Dr A. Timmis, UK.)

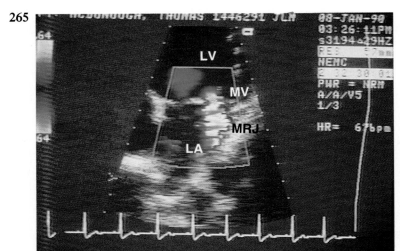

265 Apical four-chamber view (two-dimensional echoes with colour flow Doppler), showing a mitral regurgitation jet (MRJ). This technology enables a more accurate identification of the presence of valvular dysfunction than does auscultation (LV, left ventricle; MV, mitral valve; LA, left atrium). (Courtesy of Dr D. Fulton, USA.)

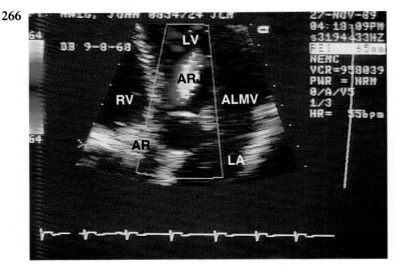

266 Apical four-chamber view (two-dimensional echoes with colour flow Doppler), showing an aortic regurgitation jet (ARJ) with the left ventricle (LV) above, and the anterior leaflet of the mitral valve (ALMV), left atrium (LA) and aortic root (AR) below. (Courtesy of Dr D. Fulton, USA.)

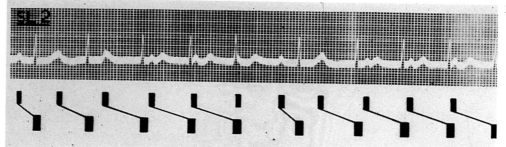

267 Wenckebach phenomenon in active carditis.

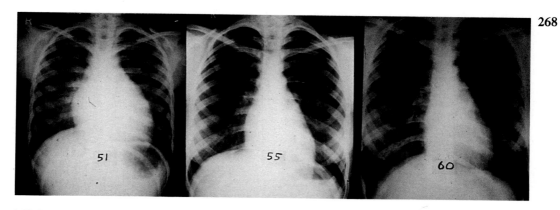

268 X-rays showing an enlarged cardiac silhouette in association with mitral systolic and aortic diastolic murmurs. A gradual improvement in the size of the heart occurred over 16 weeks; follow-up at 4 and, particularly, 9 years later showed improvement in the cardiac size culminating in, clinically, only a short mitral systolic murmur.

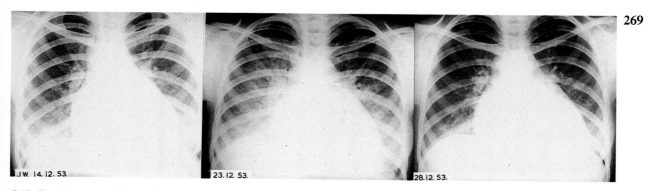

269 Persistence of a marked cardiac enlargement as a result of prolonged rheumatic activity.

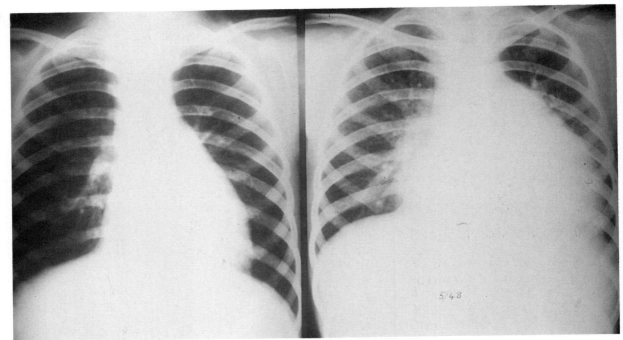

270 A child with rheumatic fever of 7 weeks' duration with pancarditis; a steady deterioration occurred, giving an increasing cardiac silhouette, and death followed 9 months from onset.

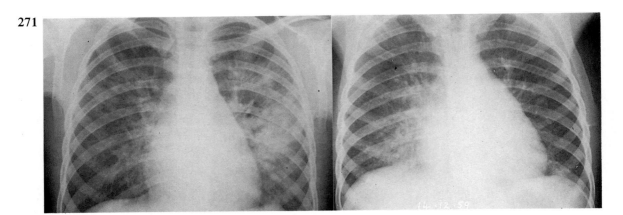

271 Acute pulmonary oedema in a boy with carditis who was being treated with high-dose salicylates. This used to be termed rheumatic pneumonia. There was a prompt response to diuretics after the introduction of corticosteroids.

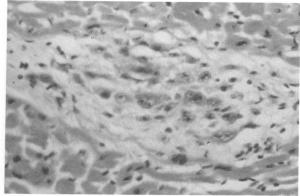

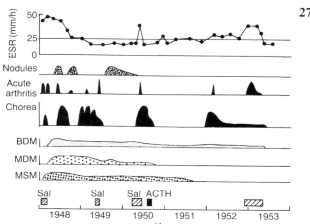

272 Typical Aschoff nodule, which is a granulomatous lesion, perivascular in position and composed of large 'owl-eyed cells', sometimes multinucleated. The large nucleus contains a prominent nucleolus, and the cytoplasm is basophilic. All are set in an oedematous base, with altered connective tissue fibres, plasma cells and lymphocytes.

273 Natural history of rheumatic fever and chorea in a patient from the early 1950s treated with only salicylate and a very short course of ACTH. (BDM, basal diastolic murmur; MDM, mitral diastolic murmur; MSM, mitral systolic murmur; Sal, salicylates.)

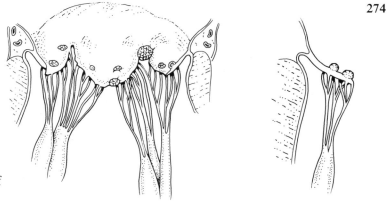

274 Diagrammatic representation of endocarditis.

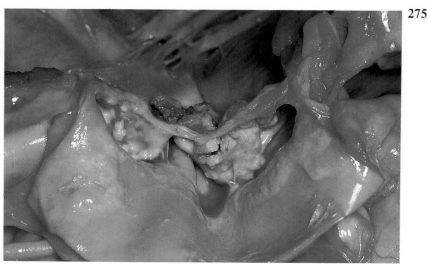

275 Calcified aortic valve.

Subacute Bacterial Endocarditis

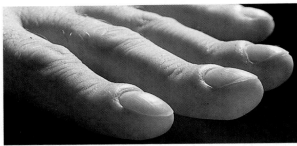

276 Early finger clubbing in a boy already known to have a cardiac lesion; blood cultures grew *Streptococcus viridans*.

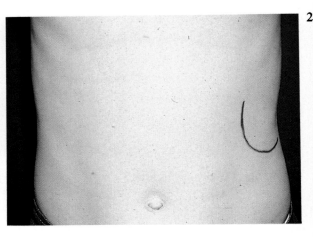

277 Palpable spleen in a child presenting with fever and known to have a cardiac lesion; investigations confirmed subacute bacterial endocarditis.

Chorea

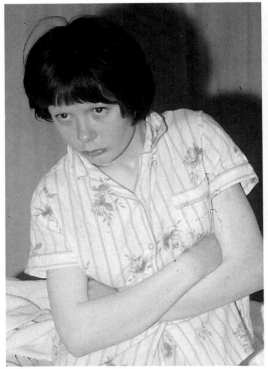

278 Chorea – note the posture of the child, who is trying to contain uncoordinated movements.

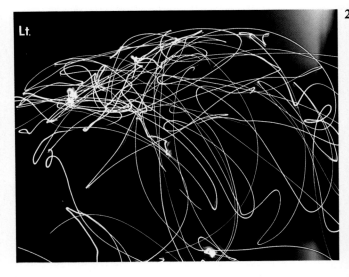

279 Chorea – light tracing over 30 seconds, with both hands extended, showing the extent of the purposeless movement.

SYSTEMIC LUPUS ERYTHEMATOSUS

General characteristics:
- Onset usually after 5 years of age
- Before puberty, female to male ratio is 3:1; after puberty it is 10:1
- Higher incidence in Blacks, Orientals, Asians, American Indians, and Latin Americans
- Can be associated with complement deficiencies C2 and C4
- Possible associations with HLA antigens HLA B8, DR2, and DR3

Clinical features:
- General malaise
- Weight loss
- Arthralgia or arthritis
- Myalgia and/or myositis
- Fever
- Mucocutaneous lesions:
    Malar rash
    Papular, vesicular or purpuric lesions
    Vasculitic skin lesions
    Alopecia
    Oral ulcers
    Photosensitivity
- Renal disease common, even at onset
- Pulmonary: pleuritis, interstitial infiltrations
- Cardiac: pericarditis, myocarditis, Libman–Sacks endocarditis
- CNS involvement: seizures; headache; psychosis
- Cerebral dysfunction: blurred vision; chorea; transverse myelitis
- Gastrointestinal involvement: hepatosplenomegaly; mesenteric arteritis; inflammatory bowel disease

Clinical features (*cont.*):
- Eye: retinitis; episcleritis; rarely, iritis
- Raynaud's phenomenon, occasionally

Investigations:
- ESR – raised
- Haemoglobin – low: autoimmune haemolytic anaemia in some; anaemia of chronic disease
- Leucopenia – mainly lymphopenia
- Thrombocytopenia in some
- IgM rheumatoid factor – may be positive
- ANA – strongly positive
- Antibodies to dsDNA usually present
- Total haemolytic complement and its components low
- Anticardiolipin antibodies and lupus anticoagulant may be present

Course and prognosis:
- Highly variable
- Relates closely to the extent and severity of systemic involvement
- Potential causes of death include infectious complications, including bacterial endocarditis
- Other problems include myocardial infarction, pulmonary fibrosis and renal failure
- Meticulous monitoring essential

Management:
- Hydroxychloroquine for skin and joints
- Corticosteroids for systemically ill patients
- Cytotoxic drugs for serious intractable disease
- Antiplatelet drugs for thrombotic episodes

Revised (Tan *et al.*, 1982) Criteria for the Classification of Systemic Lupus Erythematosus

A person shall be said to have systemic lupus erythematosus if any four or more of 11 criteria are present:

1. Malar rash
2. Discoid rash
3. Photosensitivity
4. Oral ulcers
5. Arthritis
6. Serositis:
    (a) Pleuritis
    OR
    (b) Pericarditis
7. Renal disorder:
    (a) Persistent proteinuria
        > 0.5g/day
    OR
    (b) Cellular casts
8. Neurological disorder:
    (a) Seizures
    OR
    (b) Psychosis
9. Haematological disorder:
    (a) Haemolytic anaemia
    OR
    (b) Leucopenia
    OR
    (c) Lymphopenia
    OR
    (d) Thrombocytopenia
10. Immunological disorder:
    (a) Positive LE cell preparation
    OR
    (b) Anti-DNA: antibody to native DNA in abnormal titre
    OR
    (c) Anti-Sm: presence of antibody to Sm nuclear antigen
    OR
    (d) False positive serological test for syphilis
11. Anti-nuclear antibody:
    An abnormal titre of ANA

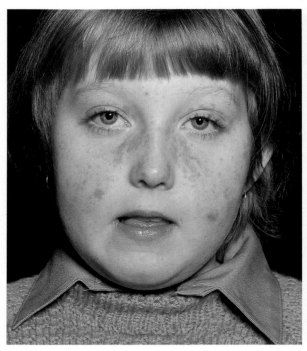

280 Typical butterfly rash in a 9-year-old Caucasian girl who presented with swelling of the proximal interphalangeal joints.

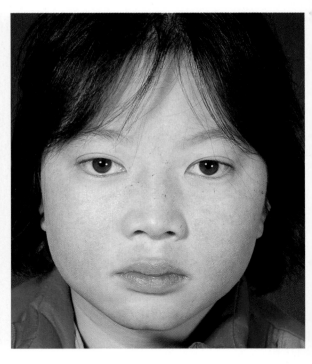

281 Extensive facial rash in a girl of Chinese extraction, which developed during an exacerbation while on corticosteroids.

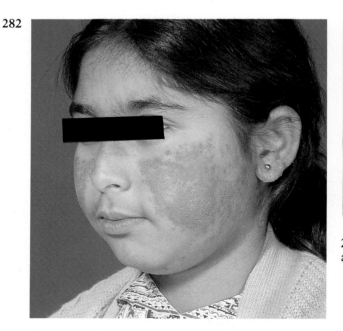

282 Acute exacerbation of a more chronic systemic lupus erythematosus rash on exposure to the sun in a young Asian girl with disease of 3 years' duration; note that the ear is also involved in the chronic discoid lesion.

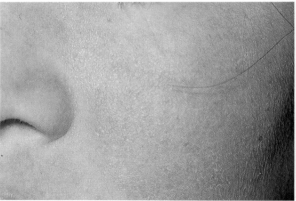

283 Close-up of patient in **281** to show the skin atrophy.

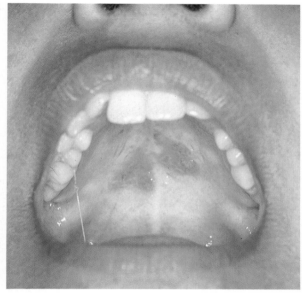

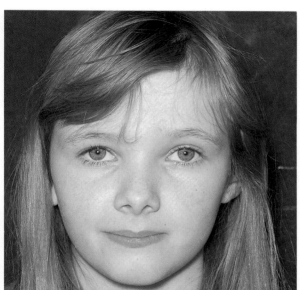

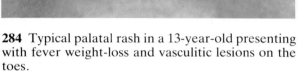

284 Typical palatal rash in a 13-year-old presenting with fever weight-loss and vasculitic lesions on the toes.

285 This 8-year-old presented with arthalgia and was noted to have hair loss and an early butterfly rash.

286 Extensive hair loss in a West Indian girl already on corticosteroids for systemic lupus erythematosus.

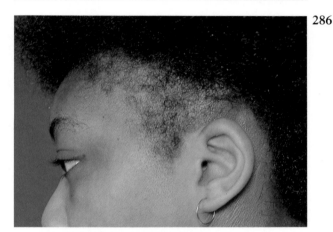

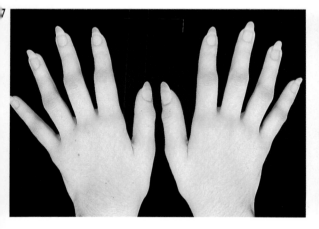

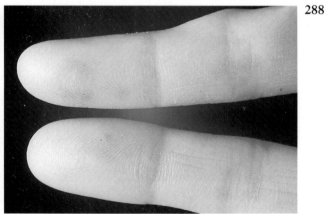

287,288 Raynaud's phenomenon; note the blanching of the finger tips in **288**.

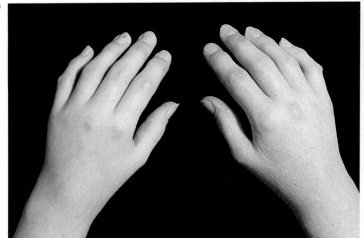

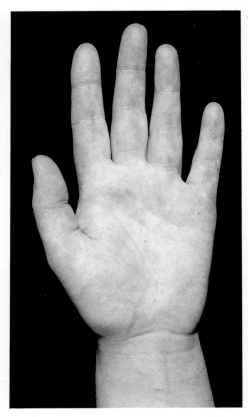

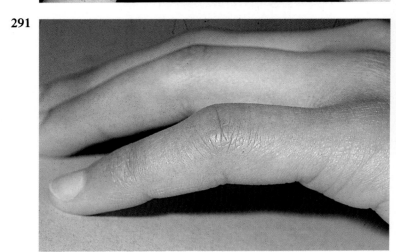

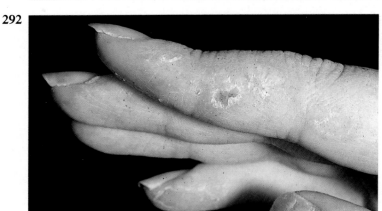

289 Acute arthritis of the hands.

290 Vasculitic lesions and chronic rash on the hand.

291 Typical chilblain lupus in a 12-year-old presenting with proximal inter-phalangeal joint pain and swelling.

292 Scaling lesions as healing of chilblain lupus occurred in a teenager.

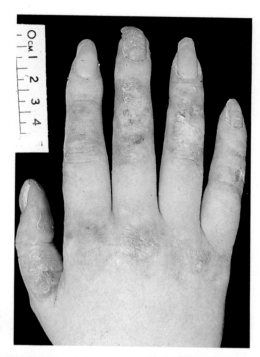

293 Scaling rash on the dorsum of the hand.

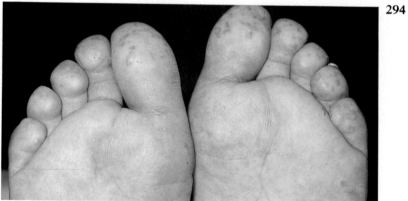

294 Extensive minor vasculitic lesions on the toes of an Indian girl.

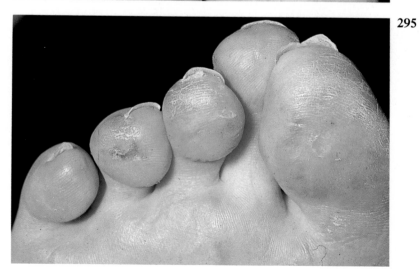

295 Close-up of the vasculitic toe lesion in a Caucasian girl.

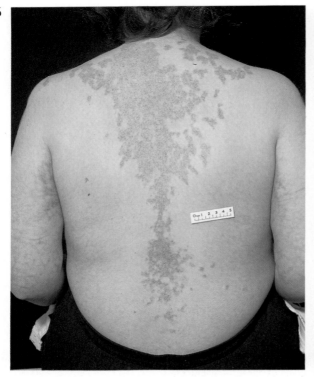

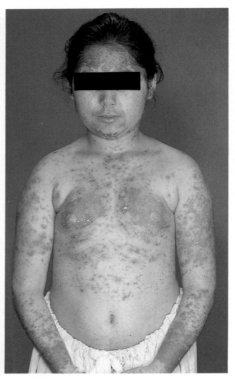

296 Chronic body rash in a Caucasian girl.

297 Extensive skin rash on the face, trunk and limbs during a systemic lupus erythematosus exacerbation.

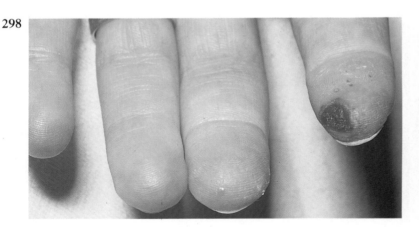

298 Vasculitic lesion in a patient suffering from Raynaud's phenomenon, causing a small area of infarction in the pulp of the finger.

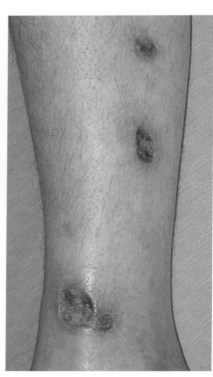

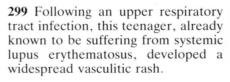

299 Following an upper respiratory tract infection, this teenager, already known to be suffering from systemic lupus erythematosus, developed a widespread vasculitic rash.

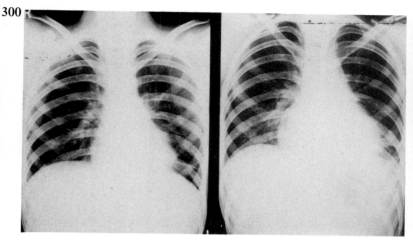

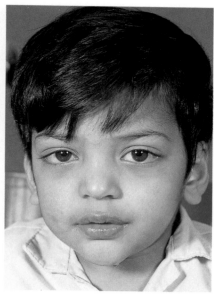

300 Pericardial effusion (in a boy aged 15) caused friction rub and ECG changes, which subsided within a month.

301 Episcleritis and blotchy rash on the face of this young Pakistani boy.

302 At presentation in 1958 this teenager had a normal chest X-ray; two years later she developed a left pleural effusion, which resolved, and then a year later a right pleural effusion; this was followed by the progressive thickening of the pleura and gradual reduction of vital capacity.

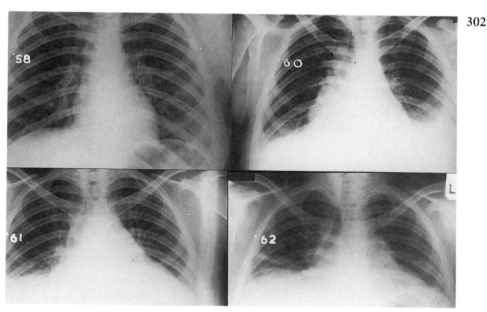

Pulmonary problems in juvenile systemic lupus erythematosus:

- Pleuritis/effusion
- Non-bacterial pneumonitis
- Discoid atelectasis
- Pulmonary haemorrhage
- Pulmonary hypertension
- Pulmonary fibrosis
- 'Shrinking lung'
- Infectious pneumonia – bacterial, fungal, or viral

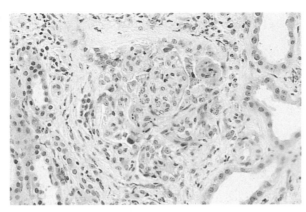

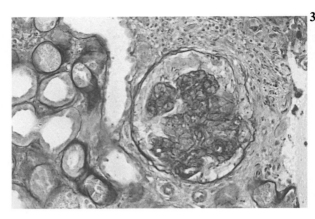

303 Renal biopsy of an Asian girl presenting with nephrotic syndrome, haematuria, and hypertension. The haematoxylin and eosin stain shows diffuse cellular proliferation. (Courtesy of Dr P. Revell, UK.)

304 The periodic acid–Schiff stain shows thickening of the glomerular basement membrane and mesangium. (Courtesy of Dr P. Revell, UK.)

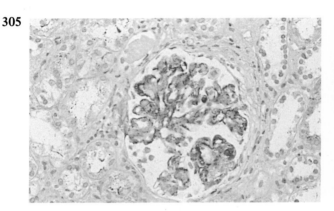

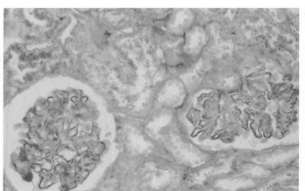

305 Heavy granular deposition of C3 along the capillary loops and in the mesangium. (Courtesy of Dr P. Revell, UK.)

306 Large granular deposits of IgG in variable positions along the capillary loops and in the mesangium. (Courtesy of Dr P. Revell, UK.)

Lupus Nephritis – Histology and Clinical Features

Type	Histology	Clinical features
1. Focal proliferative	Focal and segmental proliferation in a minority of glomeruli; IgG and C3 in mesangium	Proteinuria in all, haematuria in some; nephrotic syndrome rare; occasional renal insufficiencies
2. Diffuse proliferative	Diffuse endothelial and mesangial thickening; wire loop lesions and crescents; granular deposits of IgG and C3	Haematuria and proteinuria in all; often nephrotic syndrome; renal insufficiency in most
3. Membranous	Thickening of glomerular basement membrane due to immune-complex deposition	Proteinuria in all, nephrotic syndrome in most
4. Mesangial (minimal change)	Normal on light microscopy; IgG and C3 in mesangium	No urinary abnormality or mild proteinuria and/or haematuria

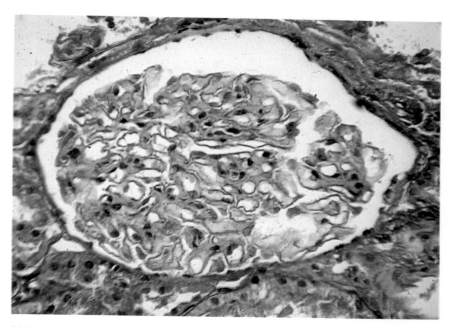

307 Focal proliferative changes with some local crescent formation in a biopsy specimen taken from a young patient presenting as having polyarthritis, but who was found to have slight proteinuria and normal renal function.

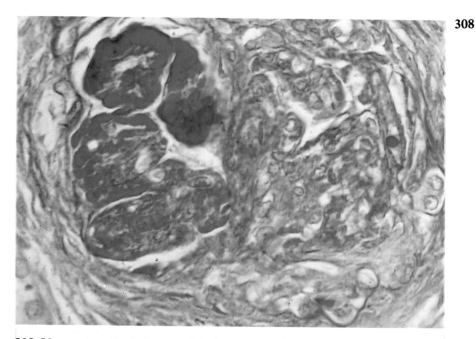

308 Very extensive diffuse proliferative changes with marked damage to the kidneys in a young patient with a rapidly progressive renal disease, which caused death 2 years from her first symptoms.

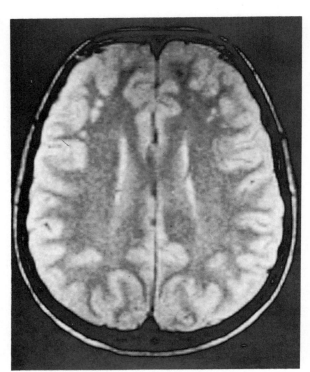

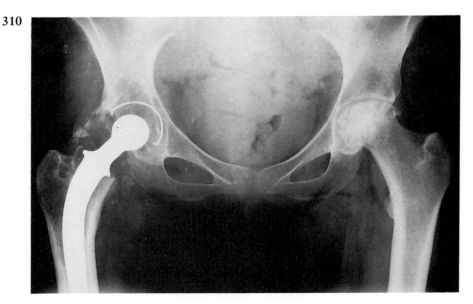

309

Central Nervous System Involvement in Systemic Lupus Erythematosus

Headache
Convulsions
Coma: Pseudo-tumour cerebri
　　　　 Aseptic meningitis
Chorea
Cranial nerve palsies
Cerebrovascular infarction
Psychosis
Behavioural disorders
Intellectual deterioration
Depression
Peripheral neuropathy
Transverse myelitis

309 Magnetic resonance scanning of the brain in a young girl with systemic lupus erythematosus. The white areas represent previous vasculitic lesions. (Courtesy of Dr P. Rudge, UK.)

310

310 Avascular necrosis of the hips in a girl of 19 whose disease commenced when she was 11 years old. She has already undergone total replacement arthroplasty on the right side.

NEONATAL LUPUS

General characeristics:
- Present in neonatal period, acquired transplacentally
- Associated with maternal auto-antibodies (particularly Ro/La) and with maternal lupus or Sjögren's syndrome

Clinical features:
- Rash – lesions of discoid lupus or subacute cutaneous lupus
- Congenital heart block – occasional endocardial fibroelastosis
- Thrombocytopenia
- Hepatic or pulmonary disease, haemolytic anaemia – uncommon

Investigations:
- ANA – particularly Ro/La
- Thrombocytopenia, anaemia, leukopenia
- Platelet antibodies – positive Coombs' test
- ECG

Course and prognosis:
- Cutaneous and haematologic manifestations transient
- Congenital heart block permanent
- Hepatic fibrosis occasional
- Some risk of systemic lupus erythematosus in teenage or adult years

Management therapy:
- Symptomatic for transient manifestations
- Heart block may require pacemaker

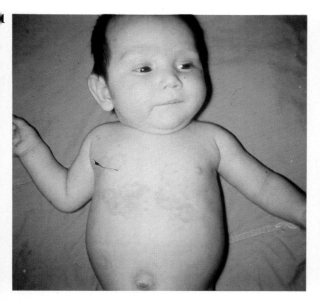
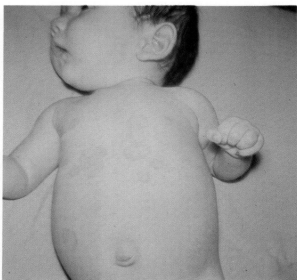

312

311,312 This baby of a mother with known lupus shows the characteristic lesions of the neonatal lupus syndrome at age 3 weeks (**311**) and at age 7 weeks (**312**). The lesions are circinate and resemble those of subacute cutaneous lupus in adults. The histology is identical to that of discoid lupus. (Courtesy of Dr J. Hodgeman, USA.)

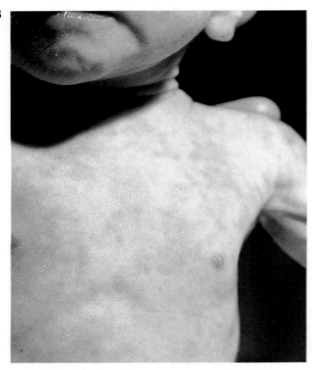

313 More extensive lesions of the neonatal lupus syndrome in a 2-week-old baby, born to a mother with known lupus erythematosus. (Courtesy of Dr J. Hodgeman, USA.)

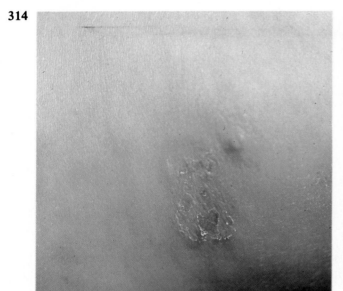

314 Close-up of neonatal lupus rash.

315 Close up of neonatal lupus rash.

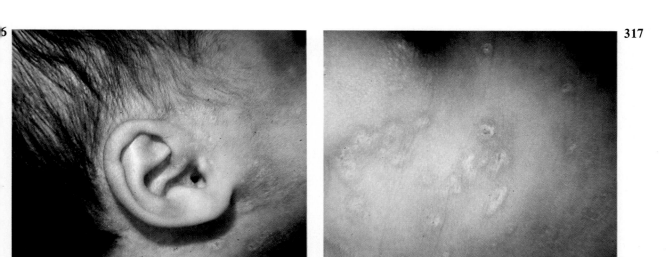

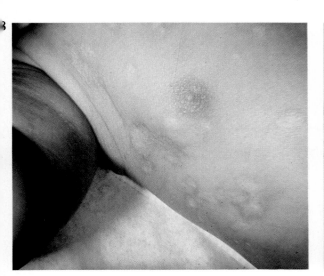

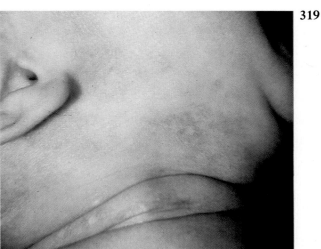

316–323 Evolution of extensive neonatal lupus rash, which had first been noted shortly after the birth of this infant born to a mother with known lupus erythematosus. The infant was found to have a positive test for antinuclear antibodies. Biopsies of the rash were consistent with discoid lupus. The infant was otherwise well. The sequence shows the development at 6 weeks (**316, 317**), 10 weeks (**318, 319**), 3 months (**320, 321**) and 9 months (**322, 323**). (Courtesy of Dr Tunnessen, USA.)

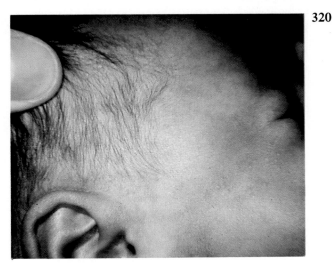

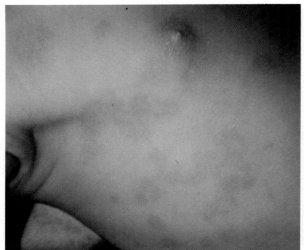

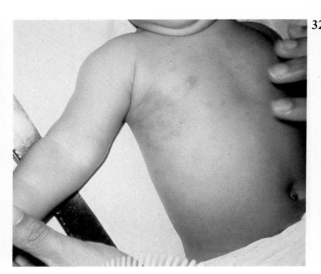

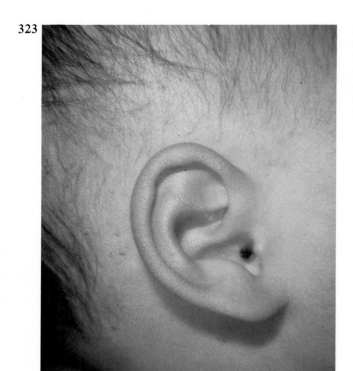

321–323 (Continued from p. 105). **321** shows fading of the discoid lesions at 3 months and **322** at 9 months. By 10 months (**323**), the infant was thriving, the discoid lesions were largely faded with only a few residual scars and telangiectasia, and the antinuclear antibody test was only trace positive. (Courtesy of Dr Tunnesen, USA.)

DERMATOMYOSITIS

General characteristics:
- Non-suppurative myositis with characteristic skin rash and vasculitis
- Girls more than boys
- Peak incidence 4–10 years of age

Clinical features:
- Muscle pain and occasional tenderness
- Muscle weakness – limb, girdle, neck, palate, swallowing
- Oedema
- Skin rash: peri-orbital heliotrope eruption and oedema
- Deep red patches over extensor surface of finger joints (Gottron's patches), elbows, knees and ankle joints
- Vasculitis and skin ulceration
- Nail fold and eyelid dilated capillaries
- Retinitis in some
- Myocarditis with arrythmias can occur
- Arthralgia/arthritis with contractures
- Limited joint mobility
- Gastrointestinal dysfunction
- Pulmonary involvement
- Calcinosis (after 1–2 years)

Investigations:
- ESR – usually normal
- Serum muscle enzymes – elevated
- EMG – shows denervation/myopathy
- Muscle biopsy shows inflammation and/or fibre necrosis and small vessel occlusive vasculitis
- ANA – positive in some

Course and prognosis:
- Variable
- Prognosis usually good with adequate treatment
- A small proportion can develop extensive muscle wasting, severe contractures and widespread calcinosis

Management:
- Gentle physiotherapy and splinting, followed by more active physiotherapy as muscle inflammation subsides
- Corticosteroids in sufficient dosage to restore function and normalize enzymes
- Cytotoxic drugs: cyclosporin, methotrexate, azathioprine, cyclophosphamide, if required
- Careful monitoring is essential, with particular attention to palate and respiratory function, as well as to possible gastrointestinal problems

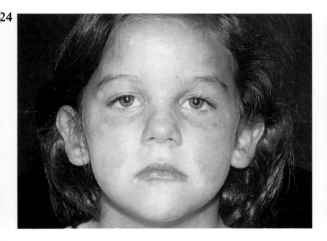

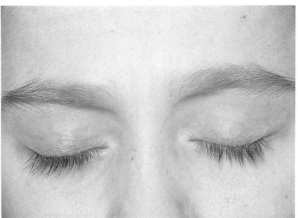

324 Mauvish rash with slight oedema around the eyelids. The evening before this rash was noticed by her mother, she had complained of pain in the calves on walking.

325 Slight oedema of the eyelids with a reddish mauve discoloration and telangiectasia.

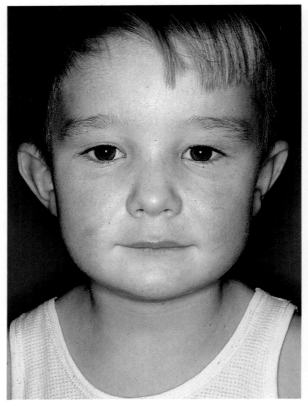

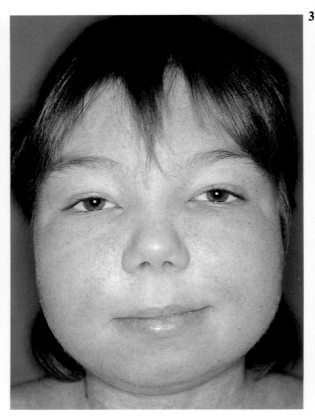

326 Typical facial rash in a 7-year-old boy.

327 This girl, already on corticosteroids for derma-tomyositis, had a severe relapse associated with a widespread erythematous rash. Note also the oedema of the eyelids and general oedematous face.

328 This child relapsed on reduction of corticoste-roids and had a widespread exfoliative rash.

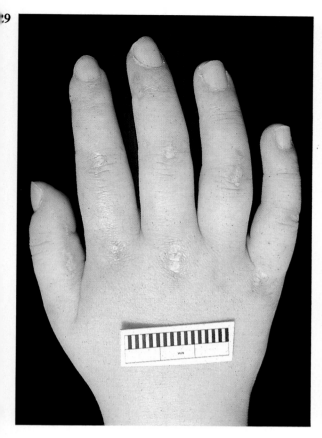 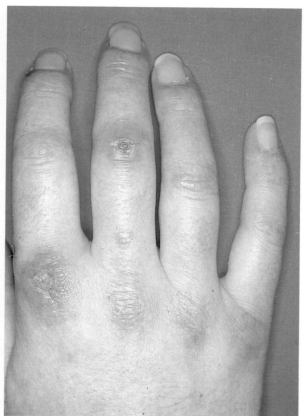

329 Hand showing widespread rash on the extensor surfaces with erythema and early collodion patches over the metacarpophalangeal joints and interphalangeal joints. Note also the slight flexion of the fingers in association with flexor tenosynovitis.

330 Acute hand showing bright rash and ulceration over proximal interphalangeal and metacarpophalangeal joints, and swelling of the fingers due to tenosynovitis.

331 Telangiectasia around the nail bed.

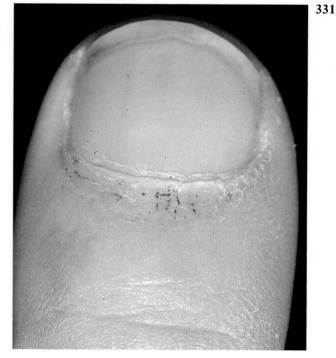

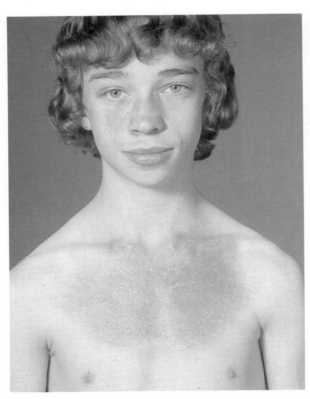

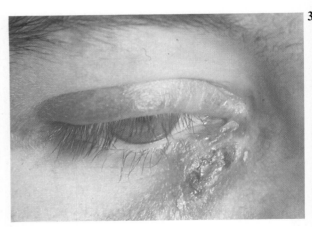

332 Chronic rash on the face and chest of a boy with long-standing low-grade dermatomyositis.

333 Acute ulceration at the side of an eye, showing an oedematous lid with early telangiectasia.

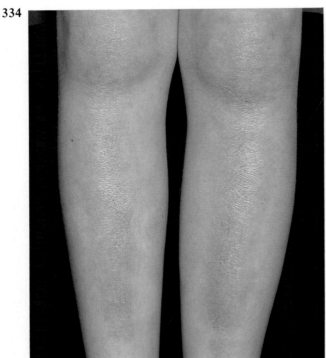

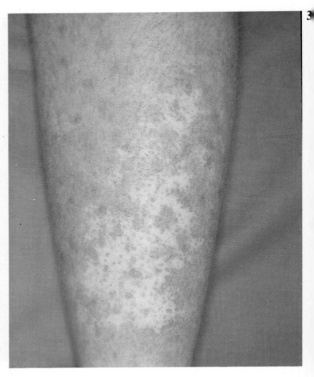

334 Extensive mauvish rash on the front of the legs in a boy who also had hand changes, but presented as stiffness of the joints.

335 An acute rash on the legs – compare with **334**.

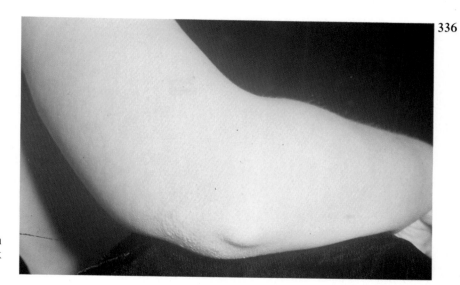

336 Acute oedema of the arm and forearm, which can mask muscle weakness.

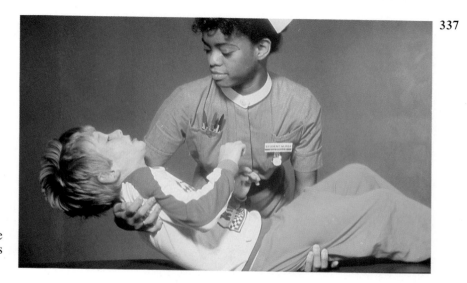

337 Muscle weakness – note the way this boy's head hangs back as he is picked up.

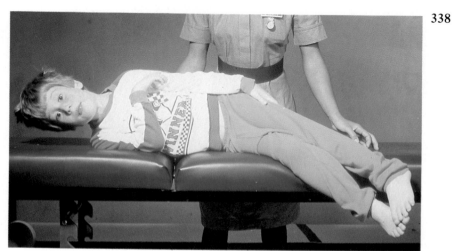

338 Inability to sit up because of muscle weakness.

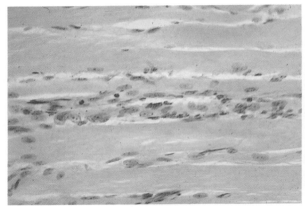

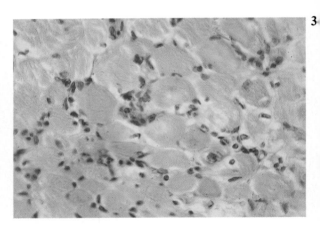

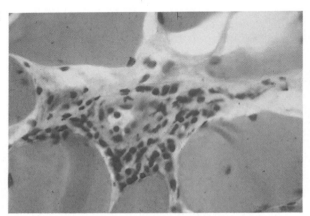

339 Longitudinal section of muscle stained with haemotoxylin and eosin (H&E), showing an inflammatory infiltrate.

340 H&E staining of a needle muscle biopsy showing variation in the size and position of nuclei.

341 Needle biopsy of muscle showing evidence of vasculitis.

342 Muscle biopsy (stained with nicotinic acid dehydrogenase–tetrazolium reductase, × 715) from a 9-year-old girl who had noted proximal muscle weakness and decreasing function for several months. She was referred as having dermatomyositis, with elevated serum muscle enzyme levels but no rash. This biopsy revealed the unexpected findings of a congenital mitochondrial myopathy (NADH coenzyme Q10 reductase mitochondrial deficiency). The finely stippled muscle fibre cells show normal mitochondria; the darkened muscle fibres with clumped mitochondria are abnormal. These histologic findings led to the appropriate diagnosis, and demonstrate the importance of muscle biopsy in patients who do not have typical disease. (Courtesy of Dr L. Adelman, USA.)

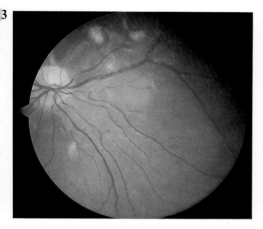

343 Retinal examination, showing cytoid bodies due to vasculitis.

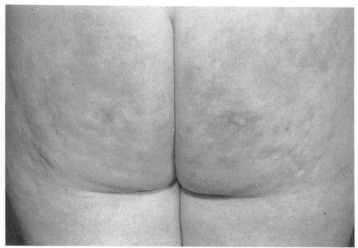

344 Mild vasculitis on the buttocks only, in an 11-year-old girl.

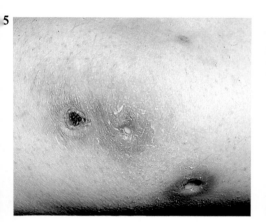

345 Severe vasculitis, causing deep ulceration of the skin of a limb.

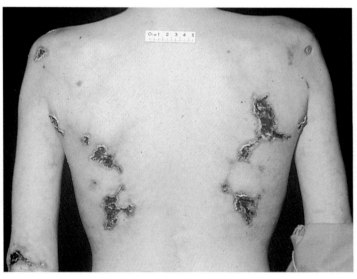

346 Extensive vasculitis, which occurred suddenly with a mild exacerbation of dermatomyositis in a teenage boy.

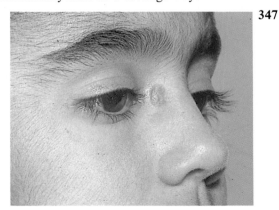

347 Healed vasculitis on the side of the nose in a young Indian patient.

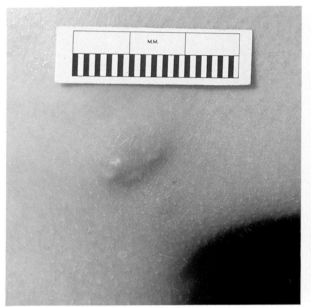

348 Nodule on knee due to calcinosis.

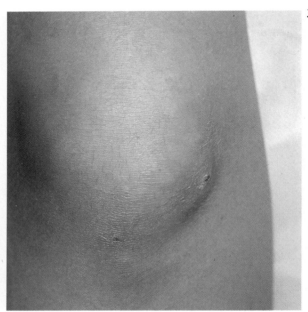

349 Calcinosis in front of the knee with some areas showing reddening and early breakdown of the skin.

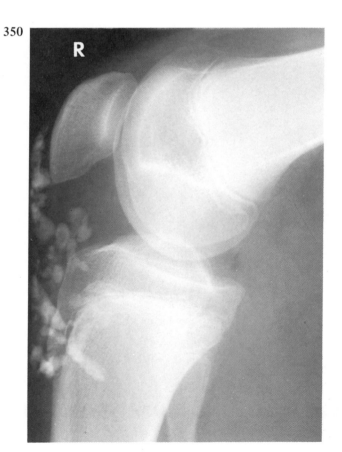

350 X-ray of subcutaneous calcinosis at the right knee.

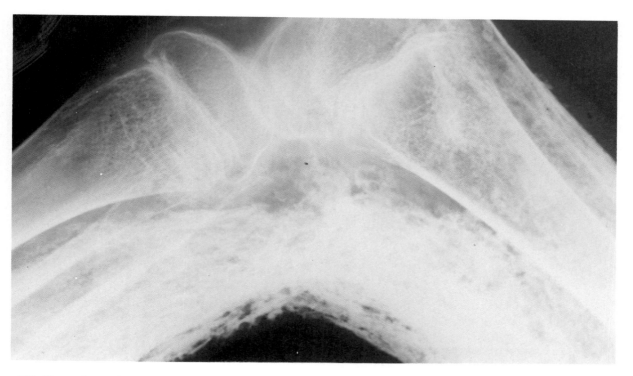

351 Extensive calcinosis in the muscles, preventing extension of the knee.

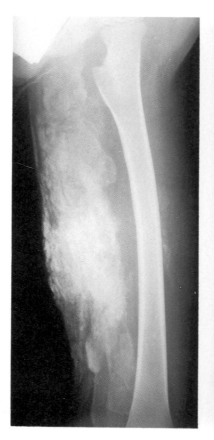

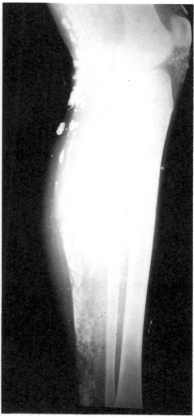

352 Calcinosis in the subcutaneous tissue and in the muscles, extending down from the thigh through the calf.

353 Both subcutaneous and intramuscular calcinosis.

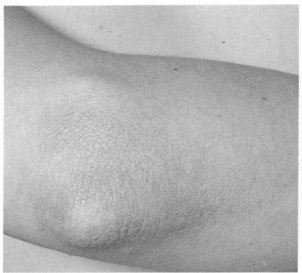

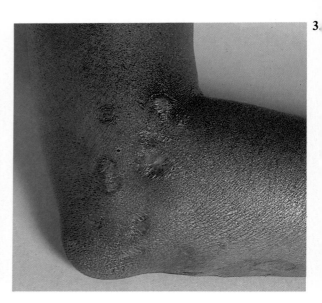

354 Acute calcinosis at the point of the elbow, which is hot, red and giving severe pain.

355 Scarring from discharging sinuses in severe calcinosis of the elbow in a Nigerian girl.

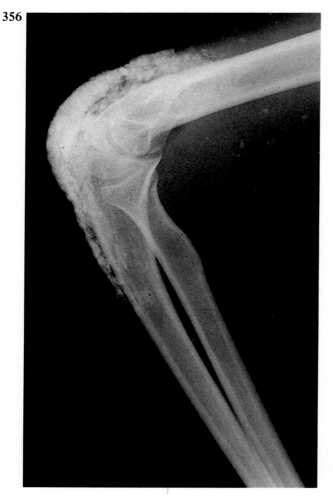

356 Extensive calcinotic lesions at the elbow without any acute symptomatology, just a gradual loss of flexion and extension.

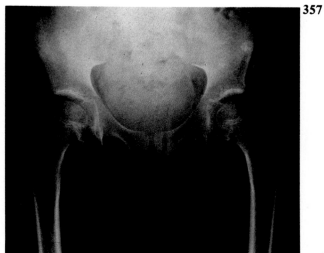

357 Calcification in the muscles around the hips.

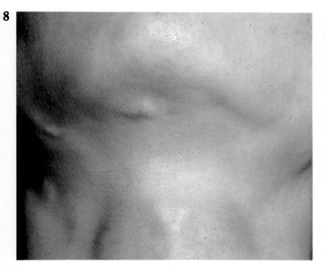

358 Subcutaneous calcific nodules under the chin.

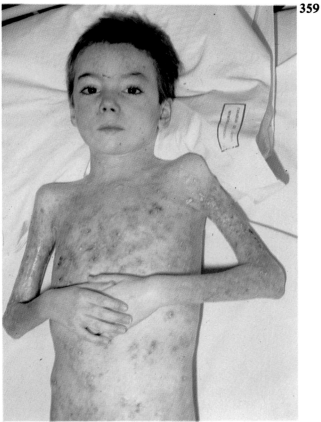

359 Chronic dermatomyositis with gross wasting, chronic rashes on the face, arms and trunk, and extensive subcutaneous calcinosis extruding through the skin.

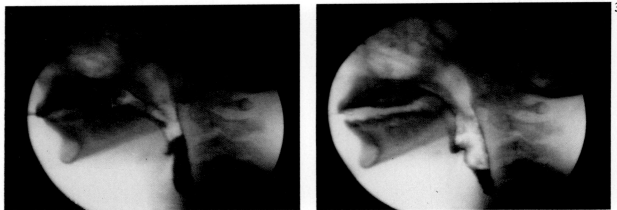

360–363 13-year-old male with dermatomyositis and swallowing difficulty. A video fluorophotometry of swallowing showed normal transport of barium across the tongue into the oropharynx. Barium then pooled in the pharynx and piriform sinuses; pharyngeal contraction was weak, with apparent failure in relaxation of the cricopharyngeal muscle. It took several further swallows to clear the pharynx of barium and some aspiration of barium into the larynx and trachea was noted. **360**, a post-swallow lateral film, shows barium pooling in pharynx and valleculae. Aspiration of barium has coated the walls of the trachea. **361** shows filling of the piriform sinuses (these do not usually fill). Barium streams down the left lateral food channel (normally, it would divide evenly around the epiglottis), consistent with a greater weakness of the left pharyngeal constrictors. A midline streak of barium is within the trachea. **362** and **363** are post-swallowing lateral views showing varying degrees of barium pooling in the pharynx. (Courtesy of Dr R. McCauley, USA.)

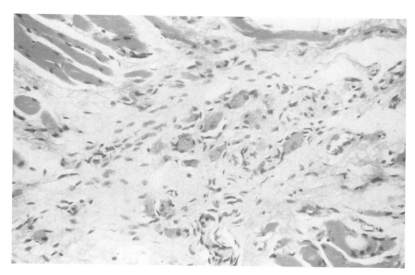

364 Histology of the oesophagus, showing destruction of the muscle fibres and lymphocyte infiltration.

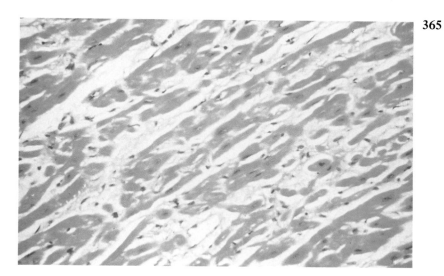

365 Myocardium of a child who died, showing gross destruction of cells. This is particularly severe – milder disease occurs in about 10%.

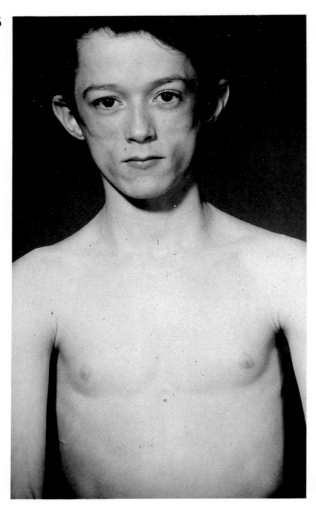

366 Fat atrophy in a child who recovered from dermatomyositis; he has hypertriglyceridaemia.

Very rarely, a pattern similar to that of dermato-myositis/scleroderma is seen as part of a graft versus host response after bone marrow transplantation. More rarely, a somewhat atypical dermatomyositis characterized by contractures and a pigmented rash is seen in viral infections in primary hypogamma-globulinaemia.

OVERLAP SYNDROME INCLUDING MIXED CONNECTIVE TISSUE DISEASE

General characteristics:
- Overlapping features of juvenile chronic arthritis/juvenile rheumatoid arthritis, systemic lupus erythematosus, systemic sclerosis, and dermatomyositis
- Affects particularly older girls

Clinical features:
- Arthritis
- Tenosynovitis – both flexor and extensor tendons of fingers, causing contractures
- Raynaud's phenomenon – common
- Myositis
- Pleuropericardial involvement
- Dysphagia
- Parotid swelling

Investigations:
- ESR – high
- Haemoglobin – often low
- White blood count – usually normal

Investigations (*cont.*):
- Platelets – can be low
- ANA – positive
- Anti-RNP antibodies in high titres indicate the designation of mixed connective tissue disease
- Anti-DNA antibodies – negative or in low titre
- IgM rheumatoid factor – occasionally positive

Course and prognosis:
- Slowly develops over years
- May evolve into other recognizable conditions, such as sclerodactyly and, later, other features of systemic sclerosis or systemic lupus erythematosus

Management:
- Mild disease managed with NSAIDs and/or antimalarials
- More severe disease may require corticosteroids, with or without a cytotoxic agent
- Careful monitoring required to detect signs of potentially serious systemic disease (e.g. nephritis)

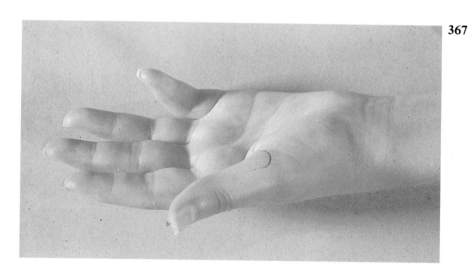

367

367 Acute carpal tunnel swelling extending onto the flexor tendons, with Raynaud's phenomenon, in a 12-year-old girl.

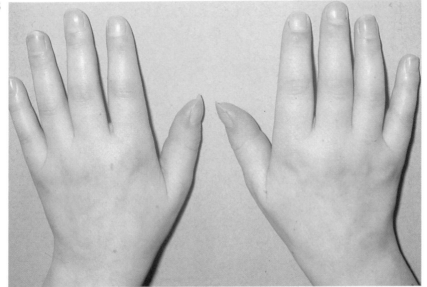

368 Marked swelling of the meta-carpophalangeal joints associated with redness and swelling of the interphalangeal joints.

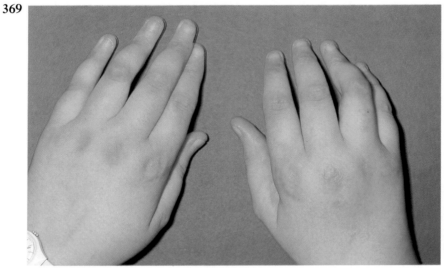

369 Swelling of the metacarpophalangeal joints with a more extensive rash on the metacarpophalangeal and proximal interphalangeal joints, mimicking dermatomyositis.

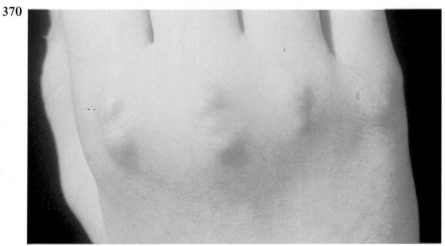

370 Small nodules along the extensor tendons.

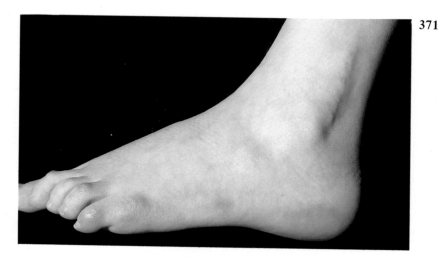

371 Extensor tendon sheath effusion around the ankle, with nodule formation alongside the foot and clawing of the toes.

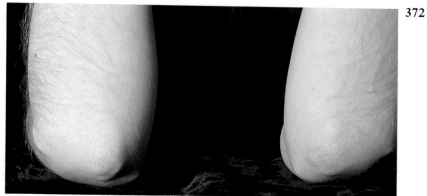

372 Multiple elbow nodules, with a histology of a bland fibrinous reaction.

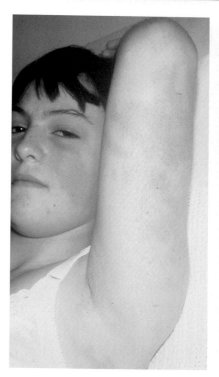

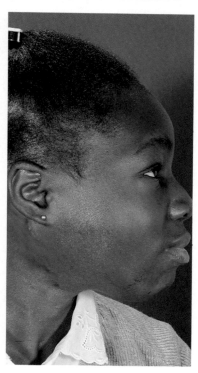

373 Nonspecific rash in a child with fever and arthralgia. Speckled ANA was present, and ENA–RNP.

374 Marked parotid swelling in a West Indian girl.

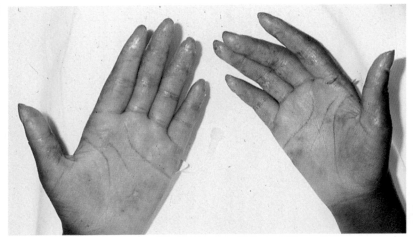

375 Flexor tenosynovitis and vasculitis in the palm.

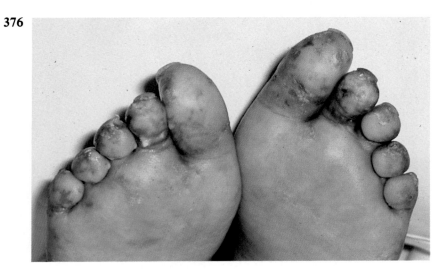

376 Vasculitis affecting toe pulps.

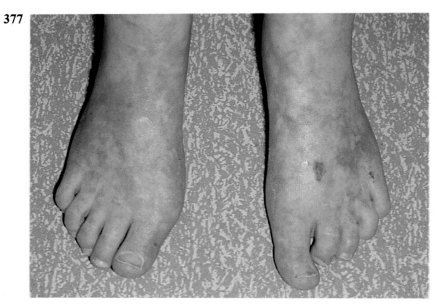

377 Vasculitis and blotchy rash on the lower legs and foot.

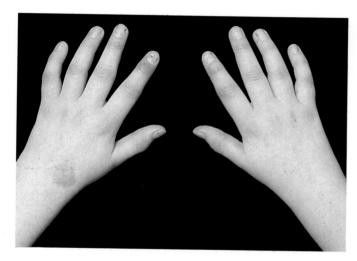

378 Hands of a girl, aged 13 years at presentation, suggestive of dermatomyositis, but with arthritis, odd rashes elsewhere and +RNP.

Female   Date of birth: 13 October 1967   **379**

RAHA < 40 ANA > 1600 Ig speckled DNA C₃C₄N

ESR 28   57   39   44 38 30 6   11

ENA   + RNP component
CPK   364   280   9   9
              Myositis
              Chest pain
          Rashes   Tight skin fingers
        Raynaud's

        Arthritis   Myocrisin

Prednisone (15/2 mg/day)

  1975   1976   1977   1978   1979   1980   1981

379 Course in an 8-year-old with arthritis, Raynaud's, variable rashes and chest pain, probably due to pericarditis and myositis, which progressed over 6 years to scleroderma.

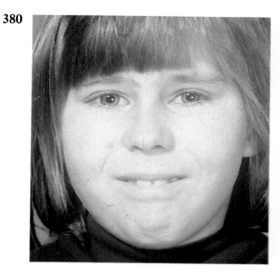

380 Recurrent parotid swelling in a young girl with synovitis of many joints.

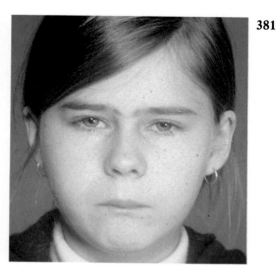

381 Same girl as in **380**, 5 years later, with puckering of skin around the mouth due to tightness; she now has classic scleroderma.

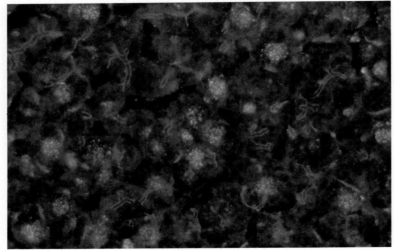

382 Speckled ANA on liver substrate.

SJÖGREN'S SYNDROME

General characteristics:
- Dry eyes (keratoconjunctivitis sicca)
- Dry mouth and carious teeth
- Parotitis
- May occur alone or in association with other rheumatic disease
- Occasional complication of renal disease or lymphoreticular malignancy

SCLERODERMA

1. *Localized* (majority of paediatric cases):
   A. Morphea:
      (i) Single patch
      (ii) Multiple patches
   B. Linear:
      (i) Face, forehead and scalp (*en coup de Sabre*)
      (ii) Limb (*en bande*)

2. *Diffuse* (systemic sclerosis)

3. *Fasciitis* with eosinophilia

Localized Scleroderma

General characteristics:
- Most common in the age range 4–10
- Sex incidence equal when young; from 7 years old females predominate

Clinical features:
- Discrete cutaneous plaques of morphea.
- Linear bands of sclerosis
  (Both the above can occur together)
- Tendon nodules/tenosynovitis
- Joint stiffness
- Arthritis in some

Investigations:
- ESR – normal and/or raised in the presence of arthritis
- Full blood count – normal
- IgM rheumatoid factor – may be positive
- ANA – positive in 60–70% cases
- Skin biopsy – shows epidermal thinning, reduction of rete pegs, collagenization of dermis and perivascular infiltration of plasma cells and lymphocytes
- Muscle biopsy – may show perivascular inflammatory infiltrates and focal muscle fibre necrosis

Course and prognosis:
- Varies widely
- Visceral involvement and progression to systemic sclerosis is very rare
- Shortening of limb due to bony hypoplasia with loss of subcutaneous fat and muscle after linear scleroderma; contractures of joints
- Rare vascular abnormalities of the brain underlying *en coup de Sabre* lesion
- Most skin lesions do not evolve beyond 3–4 years and can soften

Management:
- Physiotherapy to maintain muscle strength and range of movement
- Topical corticosteroids with occlusive wrap
- Low dose D-penicillamine
- Possible corticosteroid therapy if raised ESR occurs and arthritis is present

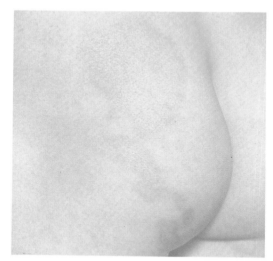

383

383 Patch of morphea on the buttock of a child who presented with stiff fingers (see **386**).

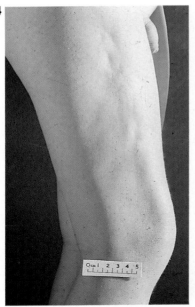

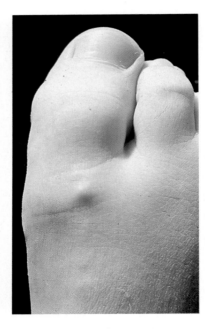

384 Linear scleroderma causing contracture of the knee.

385 Nodular lesions along the first hallux belonging to the patient in **384**, who presented with pain and contractures of joints.

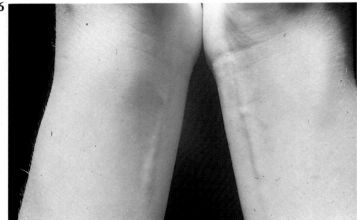

386 Nodules along the flexor tendons of the wrist in another patient presenting with joint symptoms, but who was found to have morphea (see **383**).

387 Tendon nodules along the tendon, inserting into the external malleolus, in a girl who presented with difficulty in moving the fingers and discomfort around the ankles.

388 Localized scleroderma on the back of one hand in an otherwise healthy 8-year-old girl, causing contractures of the fingers.

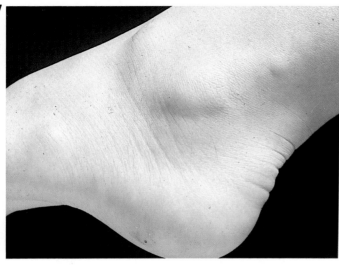

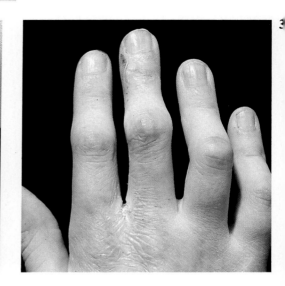

389 Localized scleroderma of the left leg in a young boy, which shows atrophy and a vasculitic element at the edge of the rash.

390 Unilateral scleroderma, affecting the forehead and face.

391 Same patient as in **390**, showing lesions on the right side: linear lesion on the right thigh and morphea on the foot. Note the slight impairment of growth of the foot in particular, and asymmetry of the body. He also has some morphea on the right side of his chest. He thus represents a mixture of morphea and linear scleroderma with synovitis.

392 Another child who has the same problems as the child in **391**, but is 5 years into the disease; note the failure in development of both arm and leg, with contracture of the hand and pigmentation of the affected leg.

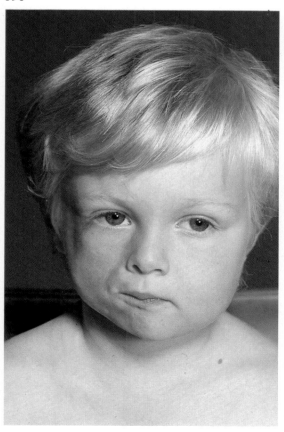

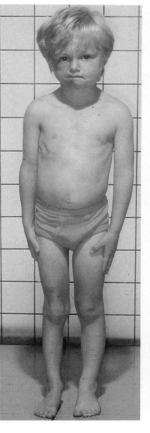

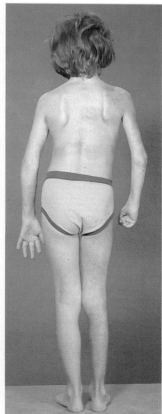

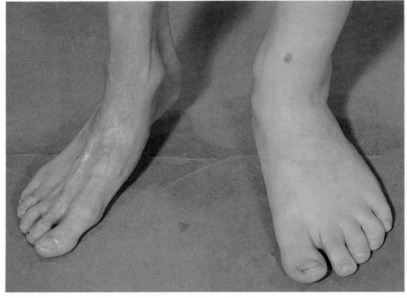

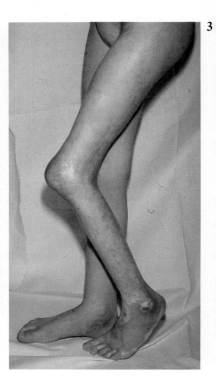

393 Morphea leading to failure in the development of the left foot.

394 Contracture of the leg due to scleroderma of the skin of the left leg in a 13-year-old.

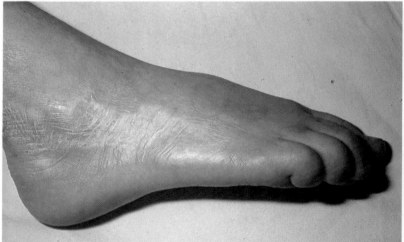

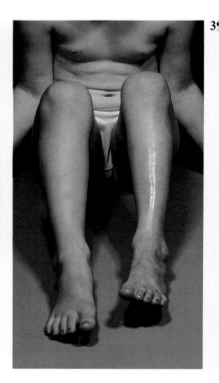

395 Localized skin scleroderma of the foot.

396 Failure in growth of the leg due to linear scleroderma.

Diffuse Scleroderma (Systemic Sclerosis)

General characteristics:
- Rare in children, but may begin as early as 3 years of age
- Female predominance

Clinical features:
- Raynaud's phenomenon, digital ulcers, sclerodactyly
- Diffuse skin thickening
- Synovitis and tenosynovitis, with creaking on movement
- Myopathy in some
- Dysphagia, malabsorption and large-bowel disturbances
- Dyspnoea secondary to fibrosing alveolitis or pulmonary hypertension
- Pericarditis
- Cardiac failure
- Hypertension; potential renal failure

Investigations:
- ESR – normal
- IgM rheumatoid factor – may be positive
- ANA – positive
- SCL 70 – may be positive

Investigations (*cont.*):
- Typical microvascular changes in skin and nail beds
- Urine – may contain protein

Course and prognosis:
- Within this group is a subgroup of teenagers who have only skin, Raynaud's and joint manifestations, who appear to have a good prognosis
- Cardiac, pulmonary or renal involvement indicate a poor prognosis
- Mortality from cardiac disease is particularly high

Management:
- Protection from the cold, and meticulous attention to the skin
- Physiotherapy to maintain strength and range of movement
- D-penicillamine – results disappointing
- Possible use of immunosuppressants in selected cases
- Possible use of corticosteroids early in the oedematous phase

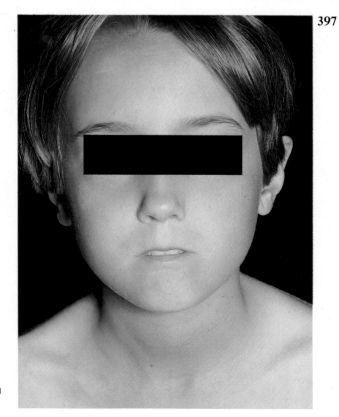

397

397 Facial appearance with pinching, discoloration and tight skin.

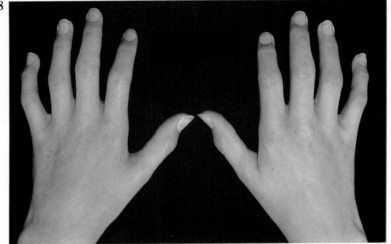

398 Contractions of the proximal interphalangeal joints, without synovitis or general discomfort.

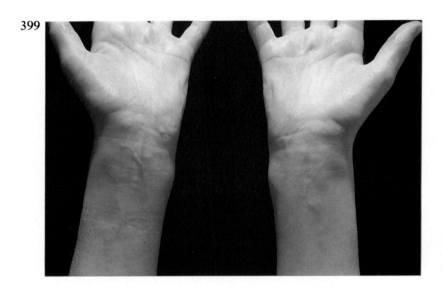

399 Extensive nodule formation along the flexor tendons on both sides.

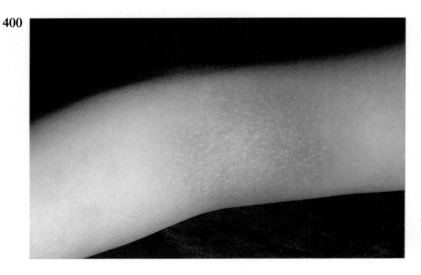

400 Pigmentation and depigmentation in a Caucasian girl; note the difficulty in extending the elbows.

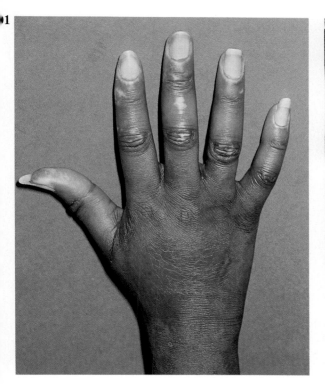

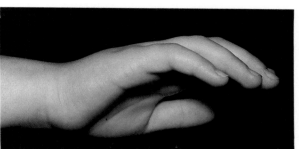

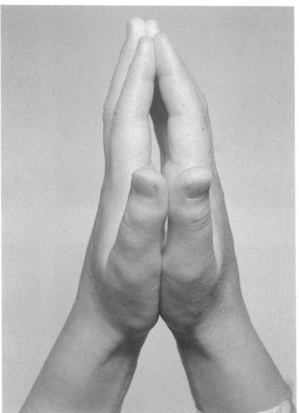

401 Extensive areas of depigmentation of the skin of the fingers.

402 Inability to extend the fingers due to flexor tenosynovitis.

403 Flexor tenosynovitis with contracture prior to gross tightening of the skin.

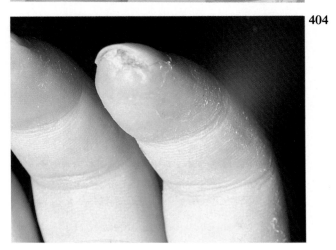

404 Vasculitic lesion causing pulp atrophy.

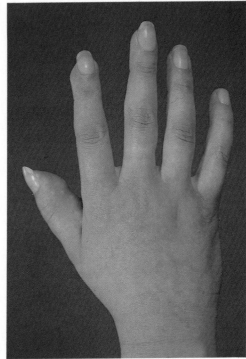

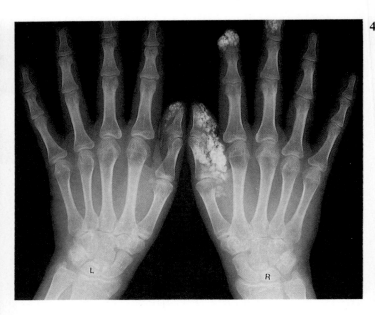

405 Lump on the thumb due to calcinosis, and pulp atrophy of the index finger in a girl with Raynaud's and early scleroderma.

406 X-ray of the case in **404** showing the extent of calcinosis in the thumb and index finger.

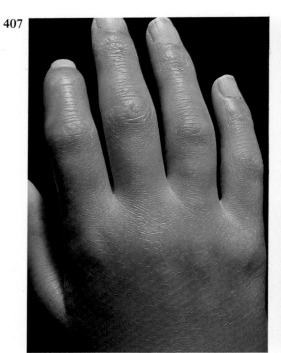

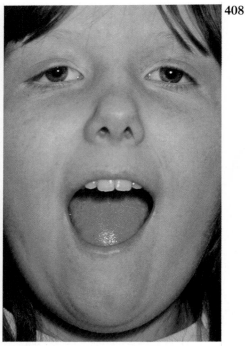

407 Marked tightening of the skin with flexion commencing at the proximal interphalangeal joints; note that this girl has lost part of the terminal phalanx of the index finger.

408 This girl has difficulty in opening her mouth, and an absence of wrinkling.

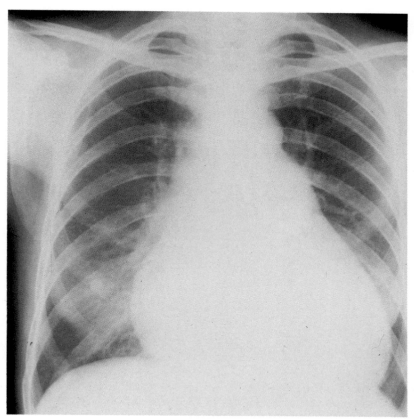

409 Early pulmonary fibrosis with
marked cardiomegaly.

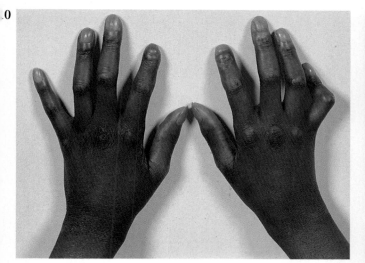

410 Contracted hands of the girl whose chest X-ray is
shown in **409**.

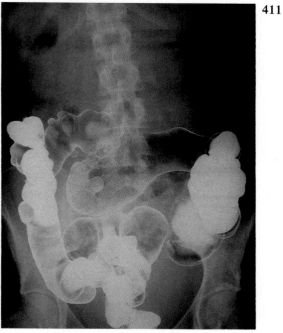

411 Barium enema showing lack of haustra-
tion.

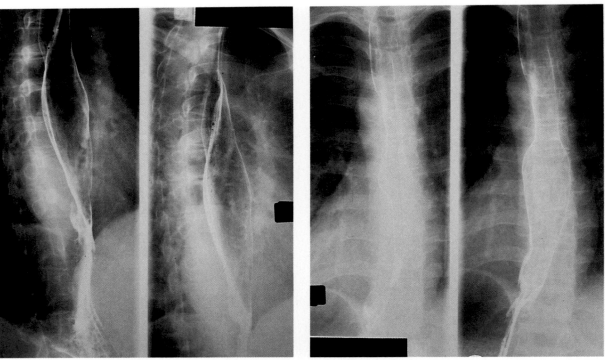

412,413 Barium swallows, showing dilatation and pooling of barium with lower constriction in a 14-year-old girl with diffuse constricting scleroderma and severe Raynaud's phenomenon; as yet there is no other visceral involvement. (Courtesy of Dr Black, UK.)

414

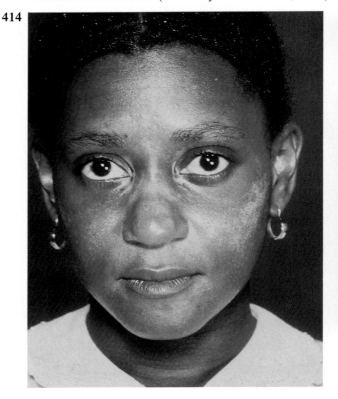

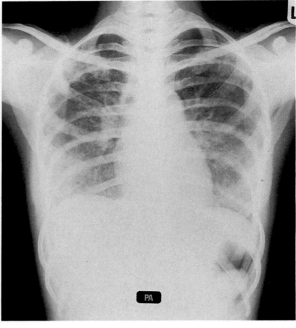

414,415 Systemic sclerosis in an adolescent with severe depigmentation (**414**) and extensive lung fibrosis (**415**), 5 years from onset.

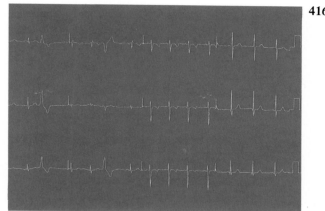

416 ECG from patient with severe myocarditis, showing extra systoles and prolonged depression of the ST segment. (Courtesy of Dr P. Follensby, University of Pittsburgh, USA.)

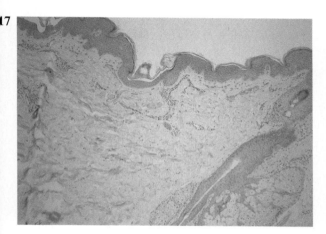

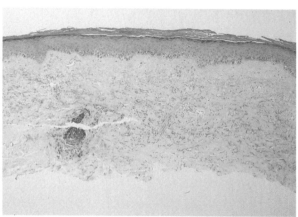

417,418 H&E stained histology of normal skin (**417**) and scleroderma (**418**) in which there is thickening and hyalinization of the dermis, as well as collagen deposition. (Courtesy of Dr Black, UK.)

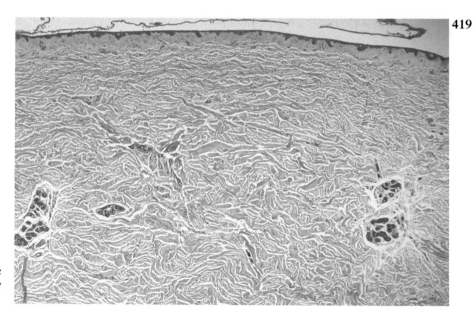

419 Note the atrophy of the skin appendages. (Courtesy of Dr Black, UK.)

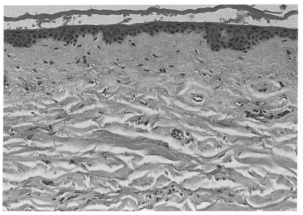

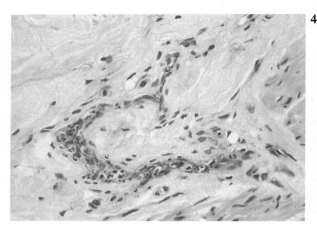

420 More thinning of the skin and extensive collagen deposition. (Courtesy of Dr Black, UK.)

421 At higher magnification, note the lymphocyte infiltration in dense collagen fibres; this type of change is particularly likely in deep linear scleroderma. (Courtesy of Dr Black, UK.)

422

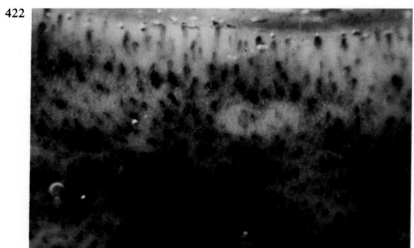

422 Normal capillaroscopy showing regular capillary loops.

423

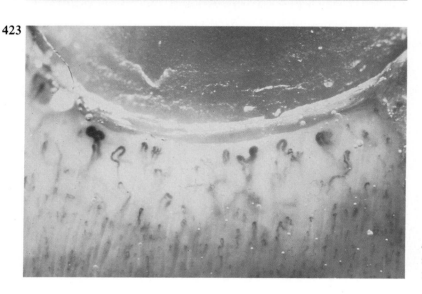

423 Capillaroscopy in scleroderma showing dilated, tortuous capillaries; note that some have dropped out.

Fasciitis with Eosinophilia

General characteristics:
- May occur in young children

Clinical features:
- Scleroderma-like swelling of a limb, often limited to the forearm or lower leg, with marked puckering of the skin
- Finger contractures
- Often arthralgia and joint contractures
- No Raynaud's phenomenon
- No systemic complications

Investigations:
- ESR – high
- Peripheral or tissue eosinophilia
- Tissue biopsy needs to include skin and fascia up to the muscle, to reveal inflammatory thickening of the deep fascia

Investigations (*cont.*):
- ANA – negative
- IgM rheumatoid factor – negative

Course and prognosis:
- Systemic involvement does not occur
- Some children have a self-limited disease with complete remission in 2–3 years
- Others develop contracture of limbs and later morphea or linear scleroderma

Management:
- Responds to high dose corticosteroids, but may relapse
- Appropriate physiotherapy to maintain function

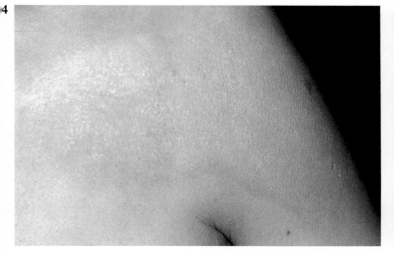

424 Morphea in a boy who presented with general stiffness and difficulty in moving.

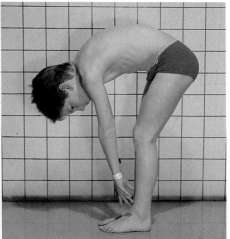

425 Same boy as in **424**, with difficulty in bending down; note the contracted knees and inability to fully flex the hips. He had a high ESR and marked eosinophilia, and was thought to have a fasciitis with eosinophilia.

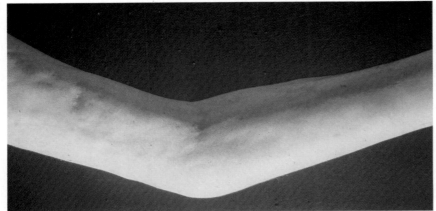

426 A more typical appearance of fasciitis with eosinophilia in a teenage girl; note the puckering and tethering of the skin, with a rivulet appearance along the upper arm and forearm. The hand was completely normal.

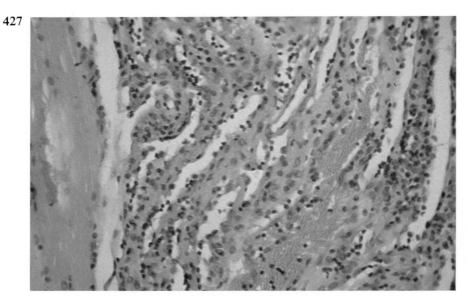

427 Histology showing fasciitis, with infiltration by lymphocytes and very few eosinophils; but the peripheral blood did show an eosinophilia.

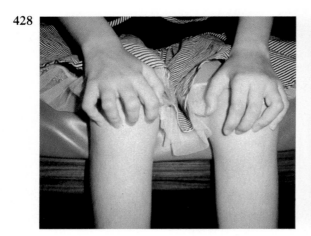
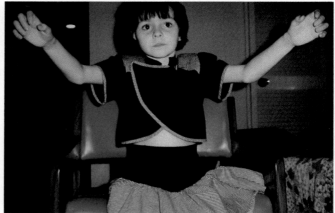

428,429 Severe finger and arm contractures in an 8-year-old girl who suffered rapidly progressive joint contractures and tightening of the soft tissues of her arms, legs, and trunk. Biopsy diagnosis was eosinophilic fasciitis.

CHILDHOOD VASCULITIS

Childhood vasculitis encompasses a wide range of clinical syndromes that are characterized by inflammatory changes in the blood vessels (American College of Rheumatology, 1990). The clinical expression of the disease and its severity depend on the type of pathological change, the site of involvement and the vessel size. The two most common forms seen in children are Henoch–Schönlein purpura and Kawasaki disease.

Henoch–Schönlein Purpura

General characteristics:
- Inflammation of small vessels, capillaries – pre- and post-capillary vessels
- May be precipitated by infection, particularly haemolytic streptococcal
- Onset generally after the age of 3 years; there is a slight male predominance

Clinical features:
- Petechiae
- Rash – urticarial lesions evolving into purpuric macules, usually on the legs, feet and buttocks
- Cutaneous nodules – particularly over the elbows and knees
- Localized areas of subcutaneous oedema that affect the forehead, spine, genitalia, hands and feet
- Arthritis – transient, involving large joints
- Gastrointestinal involvement – colicky abdominal pain and/or gastrointestinal bleeding

Clinical features (*cont.*):
- Renal involvement – nephritis, occasionally nephrosis

Investigations:
- ESR – normal or high
- Full blood count – normal
- Haematuria and/or proteinuria and/or casts
- IgA complexes in glomeruli and involved skin
- Serum IgA is often raised

Course and prognosis:
- Episodes of Henoch–Schönlein purpura are self-limiting
- Recurrences occasionally occur
- Long-term morbidity related to renal involvement

Management:
- Supportive care
- Corticosteroids in severe disease

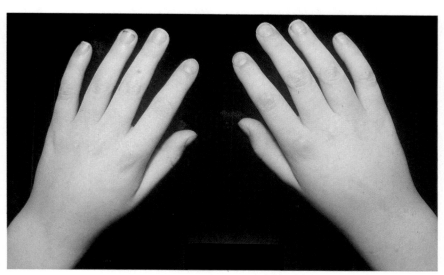

430

430 Presentation with marked swelling of one hand and slight swelling of the other in a 9-year-old boy. His rash did not develop for another 48 hours.

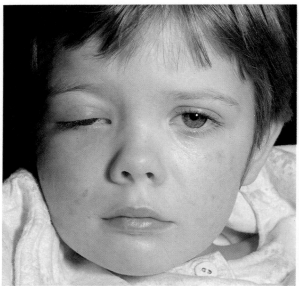

431 Unilateral oedema of the eyelid and face in a boy aged 5 years, who presented with abdominal pain and, later, a rash.

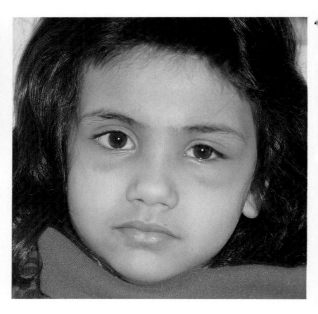

432 This little Indian girl already had a rash on her legs at the time she developed oedema around the eye.

433

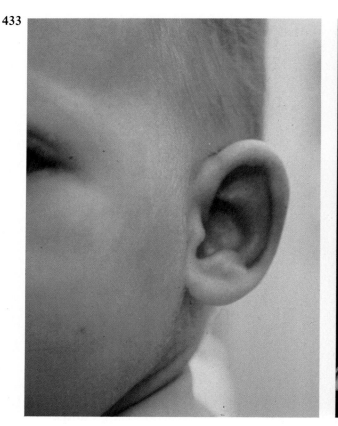

433 Vasculitic lesion on the ear.

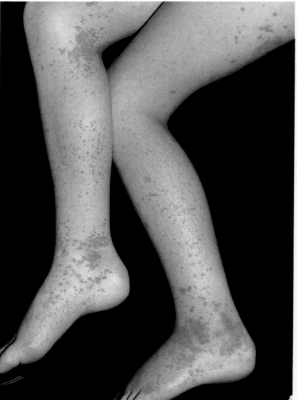

434 Extensive macular rash with purpura; note the slight oedema over the dorsum of the foot.

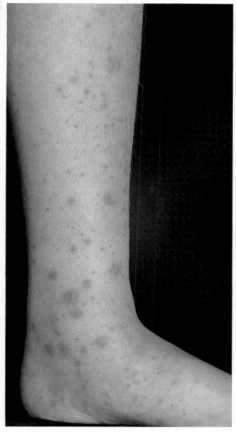

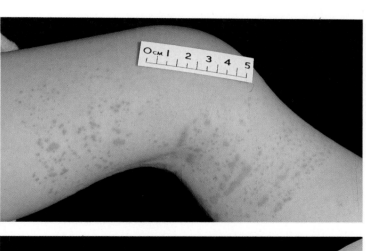

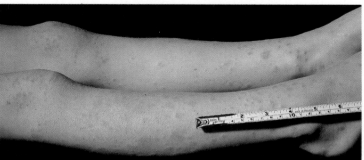

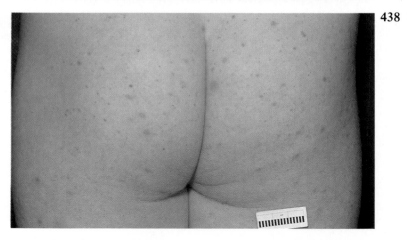

435 Extensive purpuric rash over both legs. Again, there is severe oedema on the dorsum of one foot.

436 Rash and purpura along a 4-year-old boy's leg.

437 More extensive rash of a macular type with relatively little purpura.

438 Rash on the buttock, which is a very common site.

439 Cutaneous nodules around the elbows due to capillaritis.

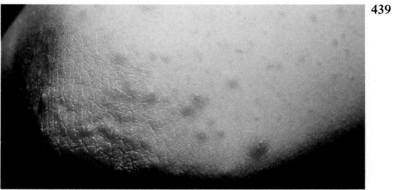

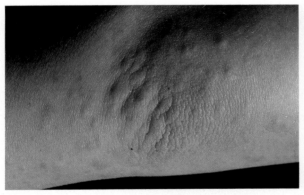

440 Papular lesions with little evidence of the purpura.

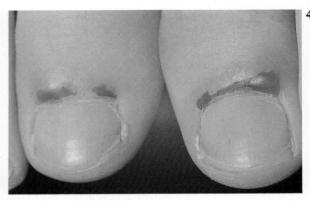

441 Lesions in the nail bed due to capillaritis.

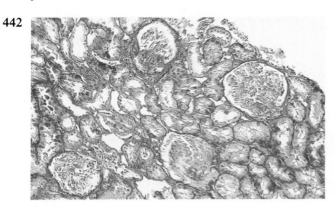

442 Acute proliferative lesion in a boy with mild Henoch–Schönlein purpura who developed a nephrotic syndrome.

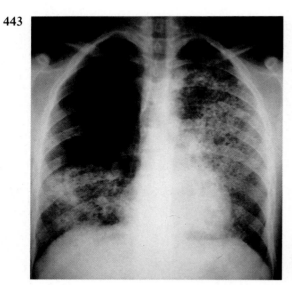

443 This boy had purpura, haematuria, arthritis and extensive pulmonary haemorrhage. (Courtesy of Dr P. White, UK.)

Kawasaki Disease (Mucocutaneous Lymph Node Syndrome)

General characteristics:
- An acute febrile disease, first described in Japan after the 1940s
- Although now seen in all racial groups throughout the world, it appears to be more common in Orientals
- Occurs in young children, even before the first birthday, and has a slight male predominance

Diagnostic criteria (Schulman *et al.*, 1984)
- Fever lasting five days or more
- Bilateral conjunctival injection
- Changes in lips and oral cavity
- Changes in extremities – reddening and oedema of palms and soles followed by desquamation
- Polymorphous erythematous rash
- Cervical lymphadenopathy

For diagnosis a fever and four features are required.

Clinical features:
  As in diagnostic criteria, plus:
- Irritability
- Pericarditis
- Valvular dysfunction
- Coronary artery disease
- Arthritis and/or arthralgia
- Gastrointestinal symptoms
- Urethritis
- Central nervous system problems – aseptic meningitis
- Iritis

Investigations:
- ESR – high
- Haemoglobin – lowered
- White blood count – raised
- Polymorph leucocytosis
- Platelets – raised
- ANA – negative
- IgM rheumatoid factor – negative
- Echocardiography – arteriograms (Suzuki *et al.*, 1990)

Course and prognosis:
- Acute and convalescent stage lasts up to 10 weeks
- Coronary aneurysms or widening in some 20% of cases
- Death due to coronary vasculitis causing myocardial infarction or rupture of an aneurysm occurs in about 1% of cases

Management:
- Supportive care
- Careful observation to detect and manage complications
- Salicylate therapy
- Intravenous gammaglobulin

- *Warning:* corticosteroid therapy is potentially dangerous

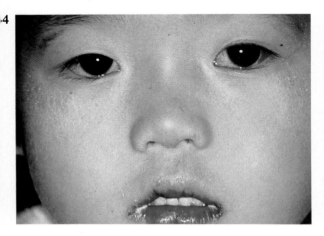

444 Face showing typical Kawasaki's disease appearance. (**444–450** courtesy of Prof. Kawasaki, Japan.)

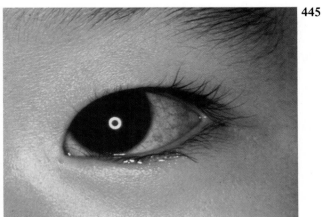

445 Eye with conjunctival injection.

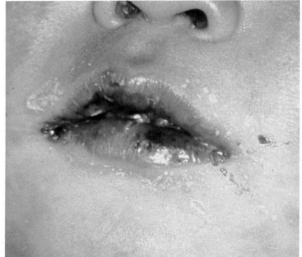

446 Mouth with swelling and cracking of lips.

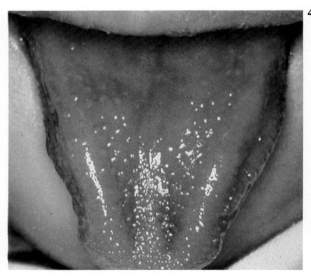

447 Tongue of a child with Kawasaki's disease.

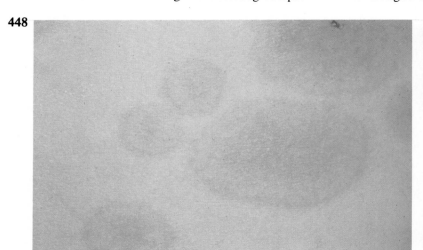

448 Typical Kawasaki rash.

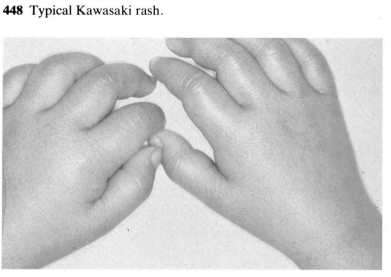

449 Enlarged cervical node in a child who also has conjunctivitis, rash, and red, cracked lips.

450 Painful, generalized swelling of the hands.

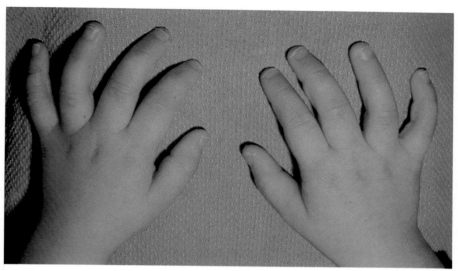

451 Swollen fingers in a 6-year-old American child who was referred with a diagnosis of JRA; in the preceding 2 weeks she had suffered a febrile illness with conjunctivitis, cervical lymphadenopathy, soreness of the lips, and polymorphic rash.

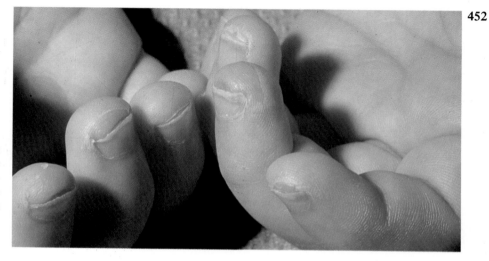

452 Close-up of the finger tips of the same patient as in **451**, showing peeling that is consistent with a diagnosis of Kawasaki disease.

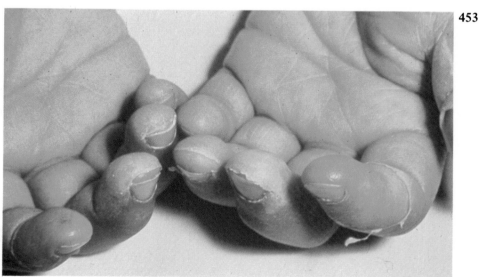

453 Peeling of the fingers of a child with Kawasaki disease. (Courtesy of Prof. Kawasaki, Japan.)

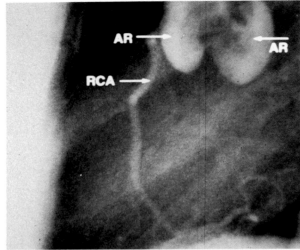

454 Aortogram showing a right coronary artery (RCA) of normal calibre (AR, aortic root). (Courtesy of Dr D. Fulton, USA.)

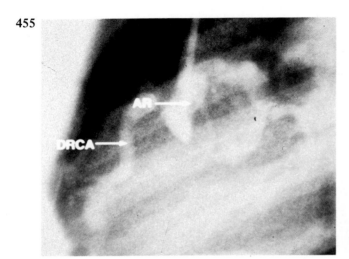

455 Aortogram showing a grossly dilated right coronary artery (DRCA; AR, aortic root). (Courtesy of Dr D. Fulton, USA.)

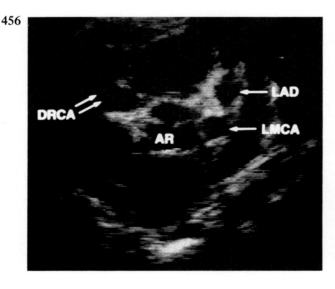

456 Short axis view of a two-dimensional echo-cardiograph showing the aortic root (AR), the dilated right coronary artery (DRCA, double arrow) and multiple aneurysms of the left main coronary artery (LMCA, single arrow) and the left anterior descending coronary artery (LAD). (Courtesy of Dr D. Fulton, USA.)

Polyarteritis

General characteristics:
- A vasculitis affecting small- to medium-sized muscular arteries in either a generalized or cutaneous form
- Age range 3–16 years with equal sex distribution

Clinical features:
- Fever
- Abdominal pain
- Arthralgia/myalgia
- Rash:
    Petechial or purpuric in the generalized form
    Tender subcutaneous nodules and livedo reticularis in the cutaneous form
- Hypertension
- Renal involvement
- Neurological disease

Investigations:
- ESR – high
- Haemoglobin – below 10g/l
- Leucocytosis
- Urinary abnormalities
- ASOT – elevated in some

Investigations (*cont.*):
- Histology – focal necrosis in small- and medium-sized arteries

Course and prognosis:
- Cutaneous form is usually benign, but relapses may occur
- Prognosis is worse in the generalized form, depending on the organ involvement

Management:
- Steroids – high dose (2mg/kg/day) in the generalized form
- Steroids and immunosuppressants for severe cases
- Penicillin prophylaxis, if streptococcal etiology is proved.

Other rare forms of vasculitis include:
- Panarteritis (polyarteritis)
- Granulomatous:
    Churg–Strauss syndrome
    Wegener's granulomatosis
- Takayasu's disease

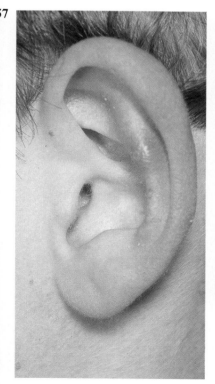

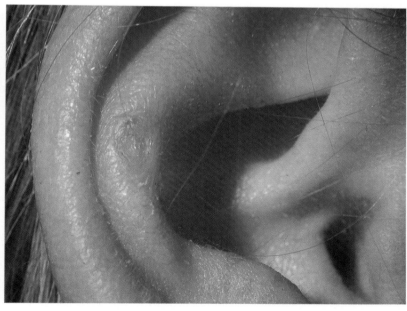

457 Lesion on the ear of a child with a high fever, arthralgia and a palpable liver. Arteriography confirmed widespread polyarteritis.

458 Close-up of another ear lesion in a child presenting with arthritis.

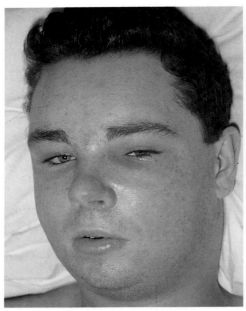

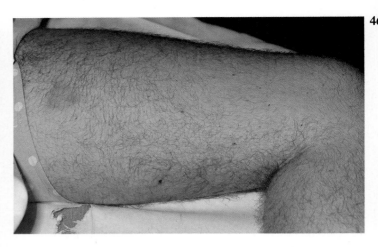

459 This adolescent boy presented with acute swelling of the face 2 weeks after a streptococcal infection.

460 Extensive rash on the limbs of the boy in **459**.

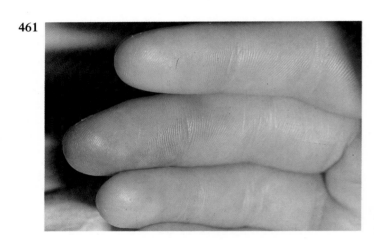

461 Vasculitic lesions of the fingers of the boy in **459**.

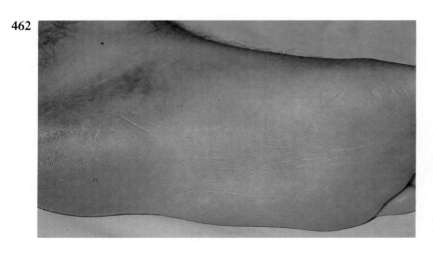

462 Palpable nodule on the foot of the boy in **459**.

463 This boy presented with a wide-spread rash, particularly on the lower limbs, following a strepto-coccal sore throat.

464 Close-up of the rash of the boy shown in **463**, which had a pattern resembling erythema ab igne.

465 This gangrenous toe of a 2-year-old was acutely associated with a high fever and general malaise and swelling of both knees.

466 Some 10 years later the patient shown in **465** had a widespread perio-steal reaction (arrowed), which aff-ected the tibiae, fibulae and femurs.

467 Lateral view of the X-rays shown in **465**.

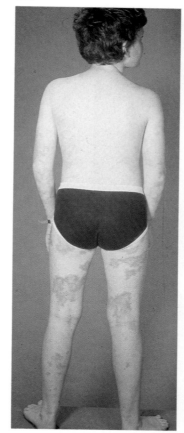

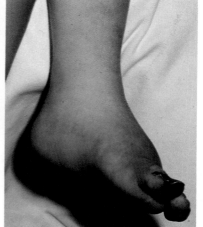

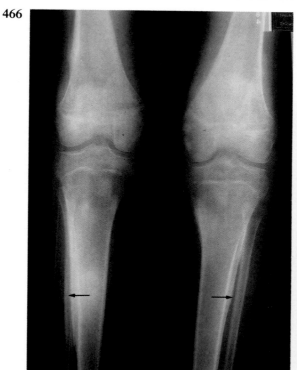

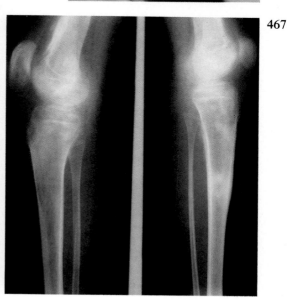

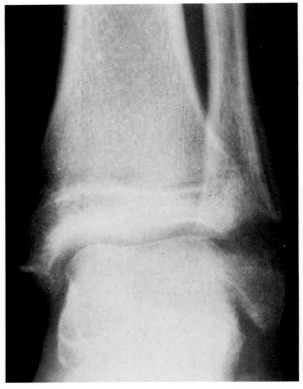

468 A boy who presented with severe pain in the ankle, associated with a rash; note the extensive periosteal reaction and osteolytic lesion along the fibula.

Leucocytoclastic Vasculitis

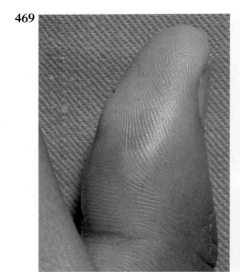

469 An acute vasculitic lesion with blanching of the thumb due to a vascular spasm in a West Indian boy.

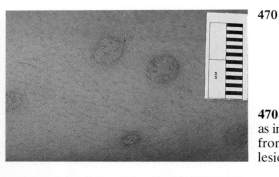

470 Arm of the same boy as in **469**, showing scarring from previous vasculitic lesions.

471 Healing lesions on dapsone.

Vasculitis with Granuloma

Churg–Strauss syndrome

General characteristics:
- A systemic necrotizing vasculitis of small arteries and veins, accompanying asthma and associated with eosinophilia

Clinical features:
- Lung involvement – asthma, transient pulmonary infiltrates
- Rash – palpable purpuras and tender subcutaneous nodules
- Peripheral neuropathy
- Renal involvement – occasionally

Wegener's granulomatosis

General characteristics:
- This also is a necrotizing granulomatous vasculitis of the upper and lower respiratory tracts, accompanied by glomerulonephritis

Clinical features:
- Pulmonary granulomata
- Destructive granulomata of the ears, nose and sinuses
- Rash

Clinical features (*cont.*):
- Glomerulonephritis
- Eye lesions

Special investigation:
- Antineutrophil cytosolic antibodies (Savage *et al.*, 1987)

Management:
- Combined therapy with steroids and cyclophosphamide

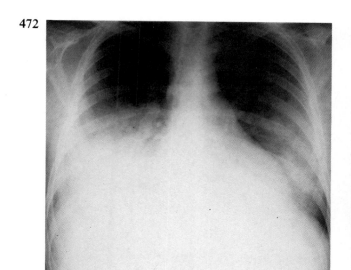

472 Wegener's granulomatosis. Chest X-ray of a 16-year-old boy who presented with acute shortness of breath and nasal stuffiness, with anaemia and proteinuria.

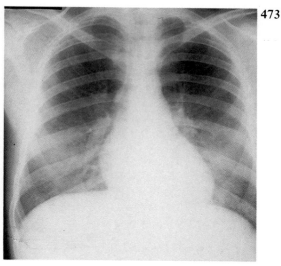

473 Chest X-ray of same patient as discussed in **472** after treatment with pulsed methyl prednisone and cyclophosphamide; note recovery.

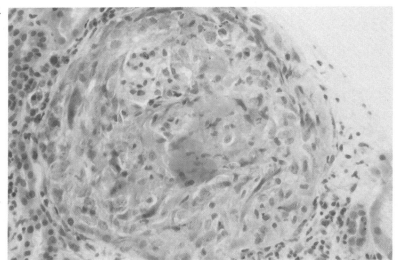

474 Renal biopsy showing glomerulitis in the patient whose X-ray is shown in **472**. (Courtesy of Dr Susan Dodd, UK.)

Behçet's Syndrome

General characteristics:
- A clinical triad of recurrent oral aphthous ulcers, recurrent genital ulcers and uveitis
- Male predominance
- High incidence in Japan, the Mediterranean and the Middle East.

Clinical features:
- Oral ulcers

Clinical features (*cont.*):
- Genital ulcers
- Severe uveitis – may lead to glaucoma and blindness
- Arthritis
- Rash – skin hypersensitivity
- Bowel involvement
- Meningoencephalitis, brain stem lesions and dementia

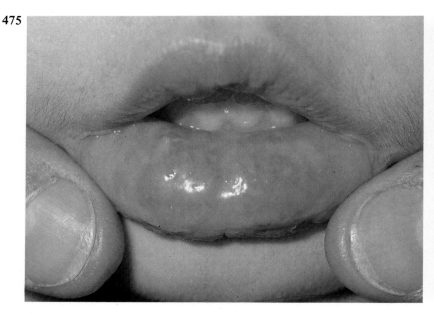

475 Ulceration of the lower lip.

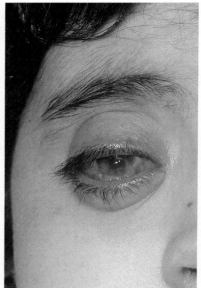

476 Severe iridocyclitis.

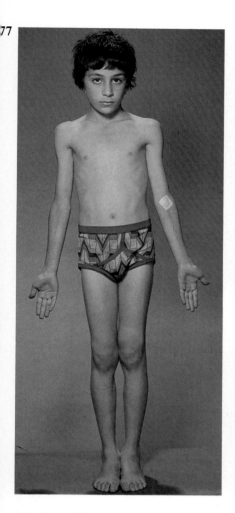

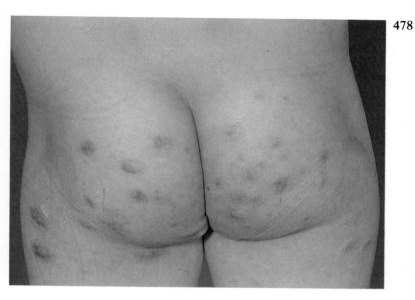

478 Sclerotic lesions on the buttock.

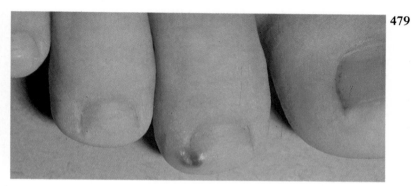

477 Synovitis of both knees in a boy with recurrent mouth and penile ulcers.

479 Vasculitic toe lesions.

Goodpasture's Syndrome

A condition of pulmonary alveolar haemorrhage and glomerulonephritis associated with antibodies reacting with glomerular and alveolar basement membranes. This can follow infections or drug exposure.

Clinical features:
- Haemostasis
- Anaemia
- Nephritis

Management:
- May respond to plasmaphoresis

Takayasu's Disease (Giant Cell Arteritis)

General characteristics:
- A panarteritis of the aorta and its large branches leading to thrombosis, stenosis or occlusion
- Primarily affects young adult women, but may occur in children
- More common in Orientals and Blacks

Clinical features:
- Claudication – in the arms and also the legs, and absent pulses
- Myalgia
- Hypertension
- Malaise
- Fever

Investigations:
- ESR – high
- Haemoglobin – low
- White blood count – neutrophil leucocytosis
- Using a combination of Doppler's and angiography it is possible to show occlusion, stenosis, or aneurysms

Course and prognosis:
- Variable

Management:
- Steroids with or without cytotoxic therapy
- Reconstructive surgery when the disease is inactive

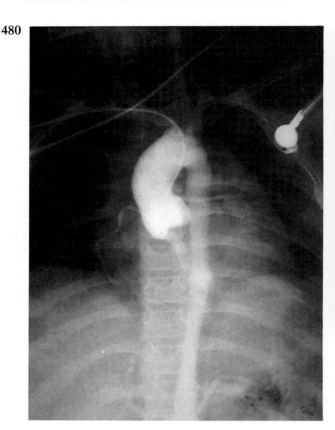

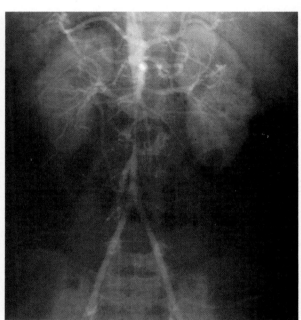

480,481 A girl who presented with recurrent fever, lower limb pains, a high ESR and a very high white count, was noted to have no hair on her legs and no femoral pulses. Arteriograms showed aortitis (**480**) and aneurysmal lesions of the renal arteries (**481**).

DIFFERENTIAL DIAGNOSIS OF CHILDHOOD RHEUMATIC DISORDERS

Despite the etiology of the majority of disorders described to date being unknown, differentiation is important because of varying complications, management and prognosis.

Note:
- Age of onset
- Sex and/or race
- Preceding illnesses
- Recent travel
- Duration and type of symptoms
- Family history

Examine:
- Overall state
- Height and weight
- Joints
- Muscle state

Examine (*cont.*):
- Skin
- Mucous membranes
- Vascular state

Remember:
- Infection
- Neoplasm
- Blood dyscrasias
- Mechanical anomalies, including injury
- Biochemical abnormalities
- Genetic and/or congenital anomalies
- Oddities *do* occur

The following illustrations have been roughly grouped under general headings, ending with a group of children who have different syndromes, some of which are not yet fully defined.

Infectious Arthritis

Viral:
- Adeno, parvo, cytomegalic, rubella, mumps, varicella

Lyme disease:
- *Borrellia burgdorferi*

Bacterial:
- Haemophilus (young), staphylococcus, streptococcus, meningococcus, gonococcus

Bacterial (*cont.*):
- Mycobacteria – both typical and atypical

Fungal:
- Blastomycosis, coccidiomycosis, cryptococcus
- *Histoplasma capsulatum.*

Other:
- Mycoplasma
- Guinea worm

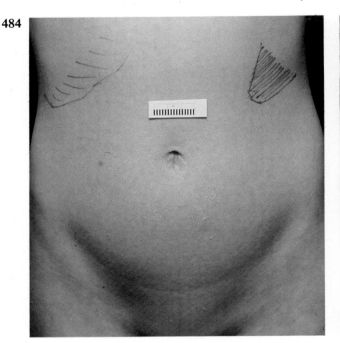

Female 6 years old							
1980 May 8	15	22	29	June 11	18	25 //	June 1981

ESR (mm/h)	110	98	98	60	24
Hb (g)	11.1	9.3	9.0	8.5	11.5
WBC	28.1	28.5	22.6	16.5	10.4
Adenoviral titres	1.2000	1.100,000		1.50,000	1.2000

482 A 14-year-old girl presented with a sore throat associated with a high fever, generalized arthralgia and bilateral swelling of the knee joints, and this somewhat diffuse blotchy rash. It was thought that she had a viral infection, and subsequent rising titres against adenovirus supported this. Her course was short, with resolution in 4 weeks.

483 Prolonged course of a younger child who was considered to be suffering from an adenoviral infection. Note that the fever is not quite as regular as that seen in systemic onset juvenile arthritis, and the rash did not coincide with the height of the fever. Neither was the rash the typical maculopapular eruption usually seen in systemic onset juvenile arthritis.

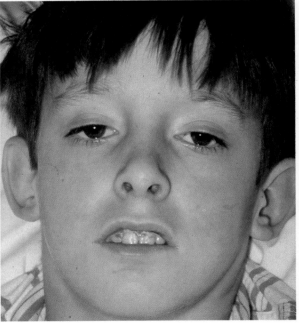

484 Note the nonspecific erythema with some desquamation and palpable spleen in a girl presenting with fever and joint symptoms, and later shown to have rising titres against Epstein–Barr virus.

485 This boy was admitted with high fever, rash and widespread arthralgia. Note the slapped cheek appearance of a parvoviral infection. (Courtesy of Dr C. Barnes, UK.)

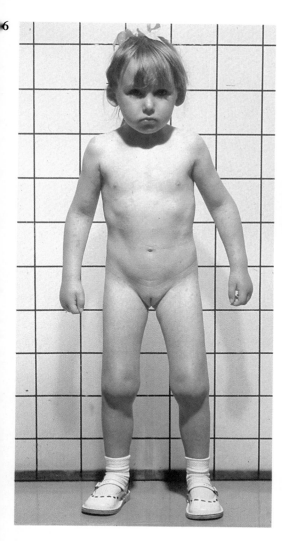

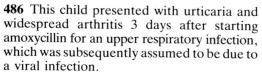

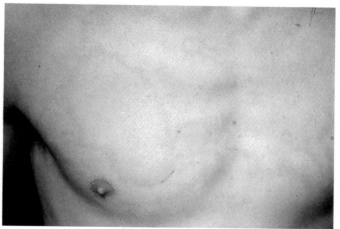

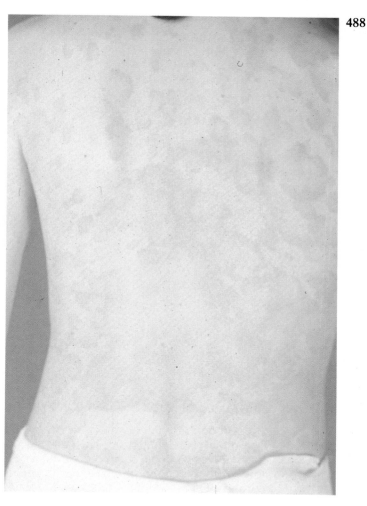

486 This child presented with urticaria and widespread arthritis 3 days after starting amoxycillin for an upper respiratory infection, which was subsequently assumed to be due to a viral infection.

487 Chronic erythema migrans following a tick bite: rising titres to *Borrellia burgdorferi*.

488 Widespread erythema multiforme in a boy found to be suffering from a *Mycoplasma pneumoniae* infection.

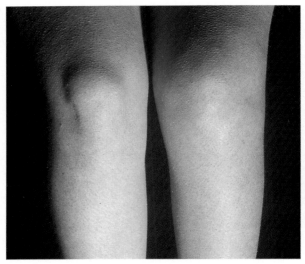

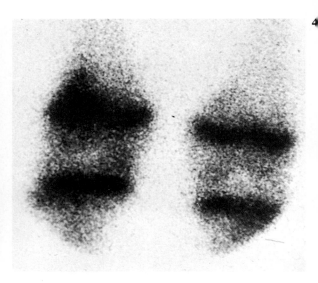

489 This 8-year-old girl presented with a hot, swollen knee, associated with rigors and high fever, 5 days after removal of a tooth associated with a dental abscess. Culture showed this to be due to beta-haemolytic streptococci.

490 Following a minor injury, this 7-year-old boy presented with a hot, swollen right knee. There was a small effusion in the knee, which was aspirated, but no organism had grown. He had local bony tenderness and the technetium bone scan showed an increased uptake. Blood cultures grew *Staphylococcus aureus*. At this point there were no radiological changes.

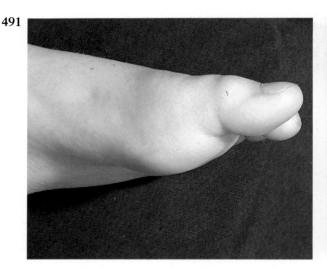

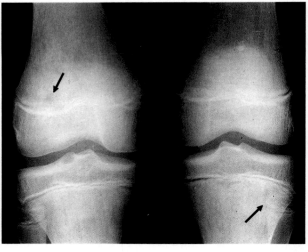

491 This 8-year-old boy presented with an acute painful, red, swollen right great toe. This was mistakenly diagnosed as gout and treated accordingly, with no benefit. When the serum uric acid returned to normal on the fourth day, reappraisal led to X-rays, which showed early periostitis on the first metatarsal, and aspiration of the joint revealed staphylococci.

492 Presentation on the fifth day as rheumatic fever, with fever and bilateral swollen knees, but also with rigors. There was marked bony tenderness at the lower end of the femur on the right and at the upper tibia on the left. Staphylococci were grown from the blood and synovial fluid, and appropriate antibiotics started. Subsequently, 21 days from the first symptom, radiological changes occurred in the original sites of tenderness (arrow).

493 Technetium bone scan showing increased uptake over the left sacroiliac joint. This 10-year-old boy complained of pain in the region of the left hip followed by dysuria. He was given antibiotics for a presumed urinary tract infection, but on the third day there was more severe pain in the left leg, with fever, and swelling of the left ankle. Antibiotics were stopped, and by the seventh day, on referral to hospital he had a very tender left sacroiliac joint. He was unable to straight-leg raise, but hip rotation was normal. Initial blood cultures for staphylococci were negative, but aspiration of the left sacroiliac joint revealed a small amount of pus from which staphylococci were subsequently grown; blood culture taken on the twelfth day, 8 days after stopping antibiotics, grew staphylococci. This difficulty in isolating the organism was presumed to be due to early administration of inappropriate antibiotics.

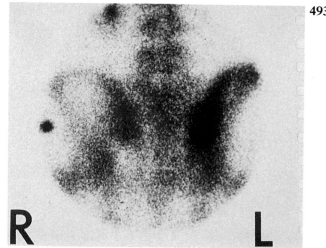

493

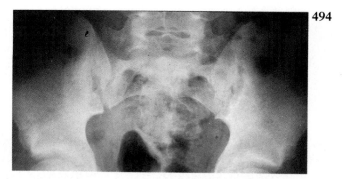

494

494 This is a radiological appearance of the sacroiliac joint of the patient discussed in **493** some 6 weeks into the illness. Subsequent bony fusion occurred.

495 A 12-year-old boy presented as rheumatic fever, with fever and widespread joint pain of 2 days' duration, but with a right shoulder that was particularly painful and swollen, and very limited in movement. In addition there was tenderness along the right clavicle.

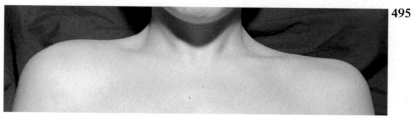

495

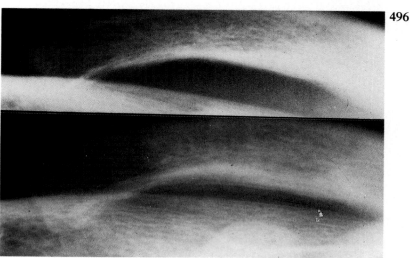

496

496 Increasing periosteal reaction of the clavicle over a 12-day period, in the patient described in **495**, despite having commenced appropriate antibiotics on the third day of illness.

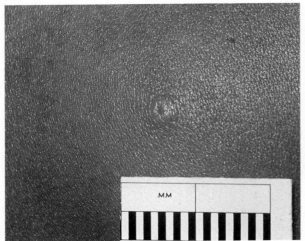

497 A 14-year-old presented with a painful swollen wrist shortly after a holiday abroad. The pustule on the skin suggested gonococcus, and this organism was obtained from the skin lesion. (On direct questioning, the girl admitted to intercourse, and a vaginal discharge of 2 days' duration for which she had not sought medical attention.)

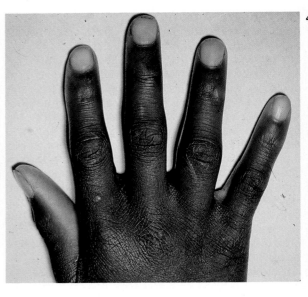

498 This 13-year-old girl appeared to be recovering from meningococcal meningitis with septicaemia when, on the fifth day, she complained of pain and swelling of her proximal interphalangeal joints. At this time her blood culture was negative.

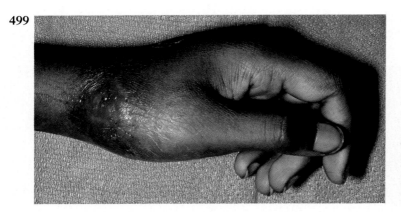

499 Painful, swollen thumb with open sinus in an adolescent Indian boy; he was Mantoux-positive and, on aspiration, tubercle bacilli were grown. (Courtesy of Dr C. Barnes, UK.)

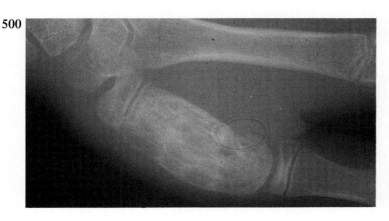

500 This shows the radiograph of the patient in **499** with severe dactylitis. (Courtesy of Dr C. Barnes, UK.)

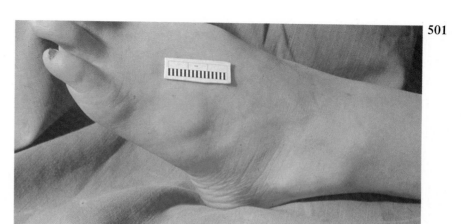

501 There was a fluctuant swelling on this adolescent Indian boy's foot, the result of tuberculosis of a metatarsal.

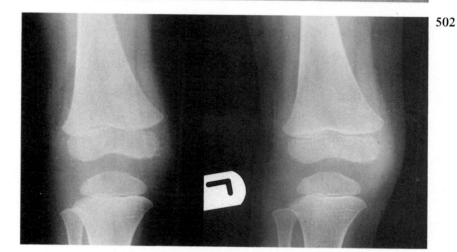

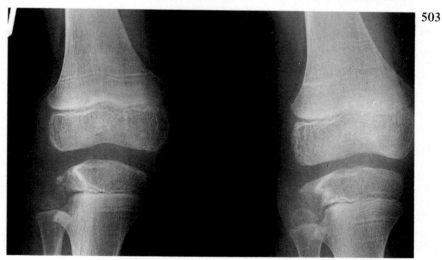

502,503 Progressive radiological changes in a girl presenting with a monarticular arthritis. Initial investigations with ESR, synovial culture, etc., were negative and the X-ray normal. One month later, local changes appeared on the tibial epiphysis and the upper end of the tibia laterally. These progressed over a 1½-year period. A further biopsy showed tubercle bacilli.

504

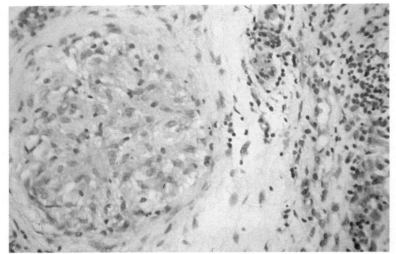

504 Histology: a granulomatous reaction with marked giant cell formation.

505

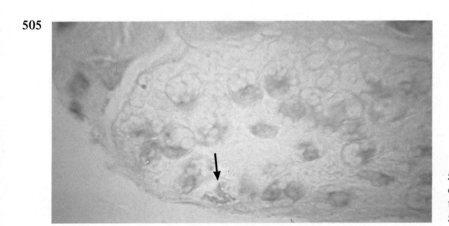

505 Close-up and specific staining of a synovial membrane shows a tubercle bacillus (arrow, see **502, 503**).

Malignancy

- Leukaemia
- Neuroblastoma
- Poorly differentiated bone tumours
- Localized tumours:
    Bone, e.g. Ewing's sarcoma
    Synovial membrane

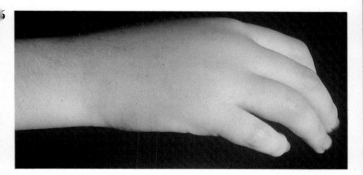

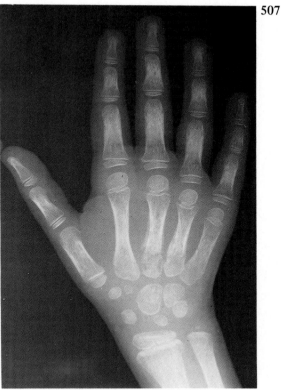

506 A 10-year-old child presented with an acute swelling of the hand with intense pain. She looked unwell and had a haemoglobin level of 9g/l.

507 X-ray of the hand in **506** showing radiolucency compatible with extensive periostitis and leukaemic infiltration at the bases of the metacarpi. Radiology is extremely useful in differentiating acute arthritis from more sinister conditions.

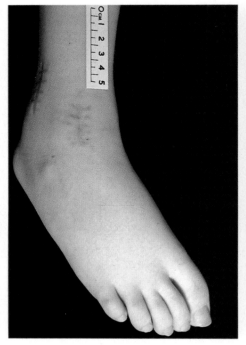

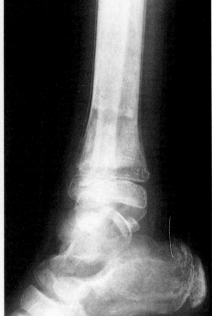

508 Swelling of the ankle and the foot; the biopsy showed only non-specific synovitis.

509 Lateral X-ray of the ankle and hind foot showing extensive leukaemic infiltration.

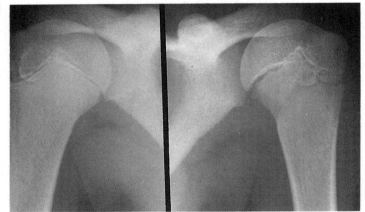

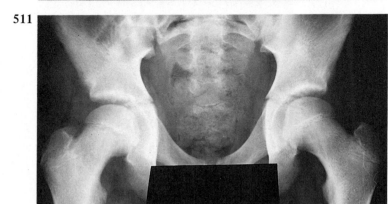

510,511 This 11½-year-old boy presented with a general malaise, fatigue and inability to keep up with his colleagues, as well as pain in the shoulders, legs and small effusions in the knees. It was initially thought to be a myositis, as he had a moderately raised creatine phosphokinase level of 480 units, but with a rather low haemoglobin level of 9.4g/l. The peripheral white count was normal, but the bone marrow confirmed the clinical suspicion of leukaemia. X-rays show extensive leukaemic infiltration in the left shoulder (**510**) and in the hip (**511**).

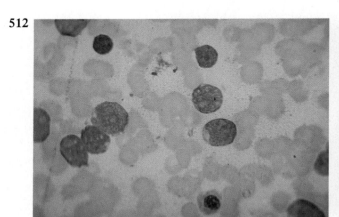

512 Bone marrow showing leukaemia.

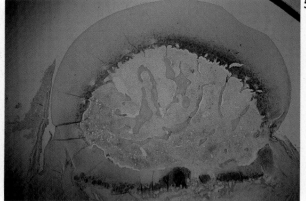

513 Section of a humeral head, showing leukaemic infiltration immediately below the epiphysis.

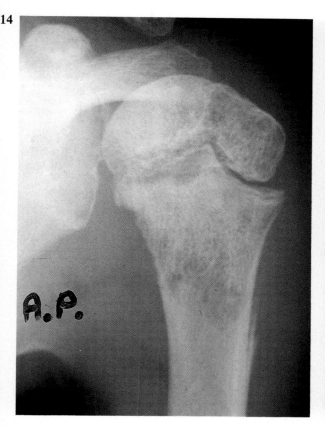

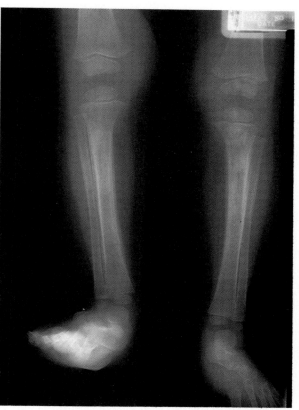

514 X-ray illustrating a child who presented as systemic juvenile arthritis with a high fever, but no rash, and intense limb pain; there was no overt synovitis. Note the extensive periosteal involvement and infiltration of both epiphysis and metaphysis. Biopsy of an enlarged cervical lymph gland confirmed the diagnosis of neuroblastoma.

515 This 15-month-old baby, who had been walking since 11 months, suddenly started to refuse to walk. There had been no marked deterioration in general health. On examination, there was a bony tenderness along the tibiae, which radiologically showed extensive infiltration and periostitis. The urine showed an increase in VMA excretion.

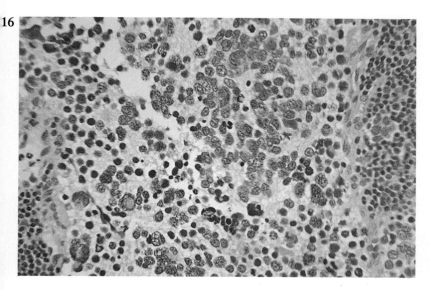

516 Lymph gland biopsy confirming a diagnosis of neuroblastoma; note the infiltrating cells.

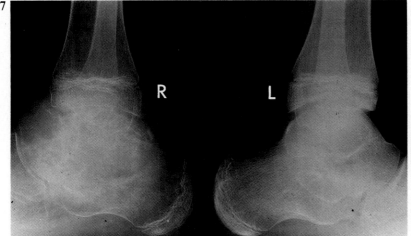

517 The boy in this X-ray presented with asymmetrical arthritis, with pain in a number of sites and gradual enlargement of the affected joints, particularly the right ankle and left shoulder. The X-ray shows dense infiltrative lesions which, on biopsy, showed undifferentiated malignant cells.

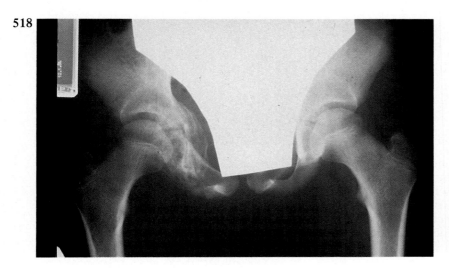

518 This 8-year-old girl was referred because of a hip problem. She had been unwell for 2 months with intermittent and now persistent pain. Her ESR was raised and her haemoglobin level was 10g/l. Biopsy of the hip had shown a nonspecific synovitis.

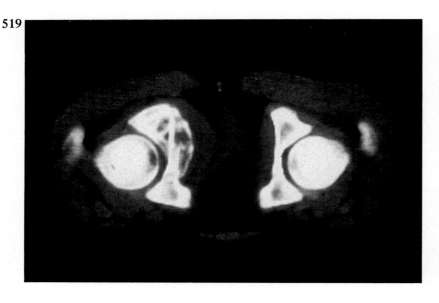

519 A CAT scan confirmed the destruction of the bone, due to a Ewing sarcoma.

Bleeding Diatheses

Haemophilia:
- Male
- Factor VIII deficiency

Christmas disease:
- Male
- Factor IX deficiency

Von Willebrand:
- Both sexes
- Factor VIII abnormal
- Rare to find bleeding into the joints, except in trauma

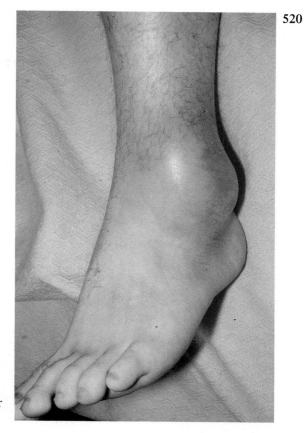

520 Bleeding over the external malleolus after minimal trauma in a boy with haemophilia.

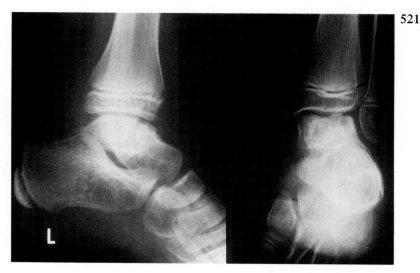

521 Destruction of the talus occurring after recurrent bleeding into the ankle in a young boy with haemophilia.

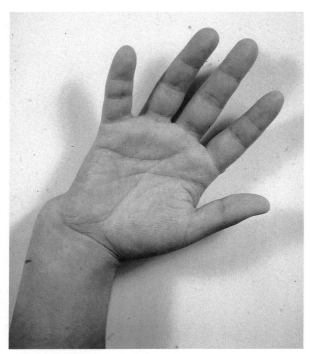

522 Recurrent bleeding into the wrist has caused contracture and loss of function in this boy with severe haemophilia. (Courtesy of Dr B. Colvin, UK.)

523

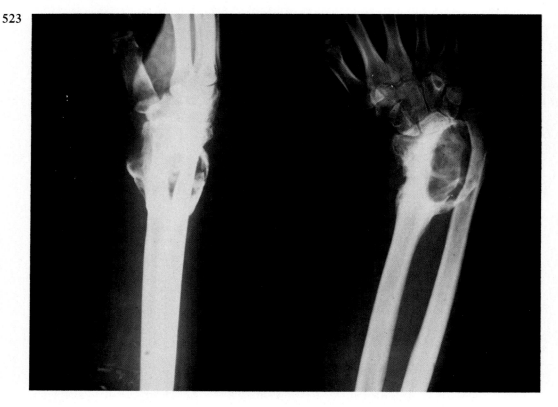

523 X-ray of the wrist of the boy shown in **522**. Recurrent bleeding into the wrist has caused progressive joint damage with narrowing of the joint space, irregular erosions, and cyst formation. (Courtesy of Dr B. Colvin, UK.)

Haemoglobinopathies

- Sickle cell disease
- Thalassaemia
- Musculoskeletal symptoms result from bone infarction and trabecular changes associated with expansion of the bone marrow due to infarction, while superimposed infection is a further problem.
- Avascular necrosis can occur in adolescents

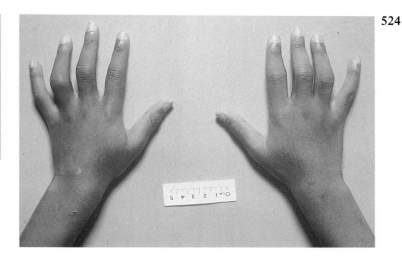

524 This 7-year-old boy had a parvoviral infection in association with a sickle cell crisis. Subsequently, he developed an acute arthritis followed by contractures of the fingers, which were shown to be the result of bone infarction.

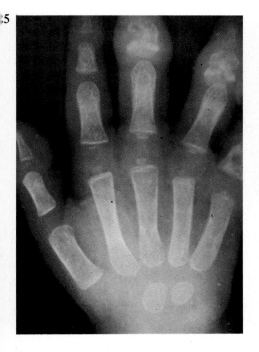

525 X-ray showing bone infarctions.

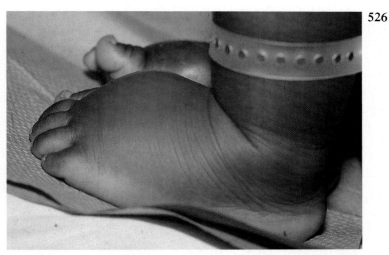

526 This represents salmonella infection in a girl of 8 months who was homozygous for sickle cell disease. Such children are particularly prone to salmonella infection, possibly due to the opsonizing activity of complement-mediated serum being defective. (Courtesy of Dr L. Tillyer, UK.)

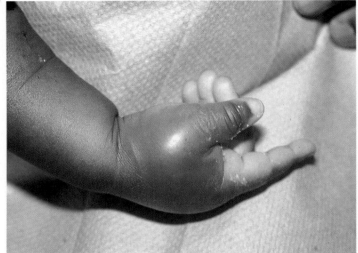

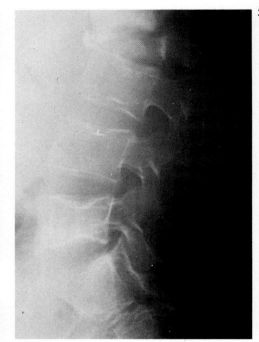

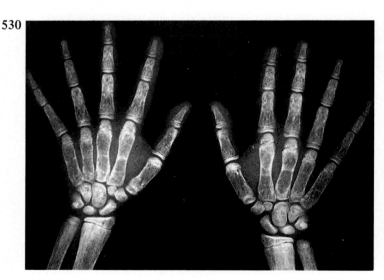

527 Hand of the child with salmonella infection described in **526**. (Courtesy of Dr L. Tillyer, UK.)

528 Spine X-ray showing a combination of the classic changes in vertebrae in sickle cell disease, with coarsening of the trabeculae and central cup-like indentations. In addition, osteomyelitis due to *Salmonella typhimurium* has caused collapse of a vertebra.

529 Blood smear showing sickle cells.

530 Thalassaemia showing generalized thinning of the bones in the hands, but no localized areas of infarction. It is beta-thalassaemia major that gives rise to the skeletal problems, but these are not a presenting feature as the disease is recognized in early life because of anaemia, splenomegaly and hepatomegaly.

Mechanical Problems

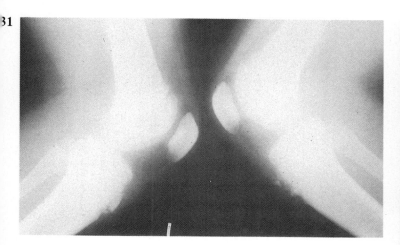

531 A girl presented with pain in her knee. It was very tender over the tibial tubercle, which is typical of Osgood–Schalatter's disease.

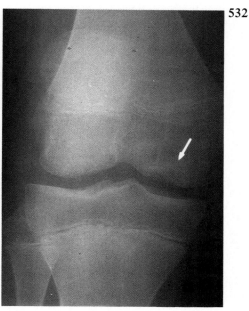

532 A boy presented with recurrent pain and swelling of the knee, which would give way from time to time; note the typical osteochondritis dissecans (arrow). Occasionally, this is multiple and affects both the knees and elbows.

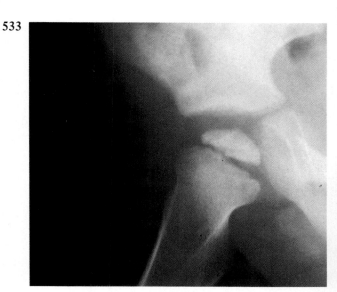

533 A young boy presented with pain in the knee, which appeared completely normal, but there was marked wasting of the quadriceps. The hip moved normally, but an X-ray showed Perthes' disease.

534 An 8-year-old girl presented with recurrent, acute pain in her hips; between recurrences she was completely normal. After six such bouts, tomography revealed an osteoid osteoma (arrowed), which had been suspected initially on a technetium scan.

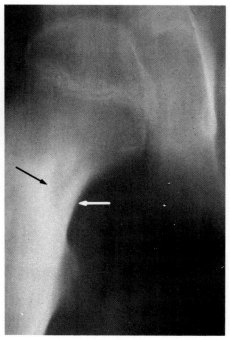

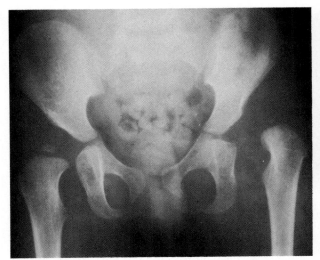

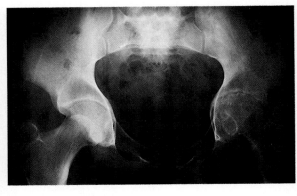

535 This baby had a congenital dislocation of the left hip, which was not spotted until difficulty in walking occurred. The mother had marked generalized hypermobility.

536 This 13-year-old adolescent boy presented with increasing pain in both hips, and with difficulty in squatting. He proved to have idiopathic protrusion, particularly marked on the left, where there is osteoporosis, presumably due to disuse.

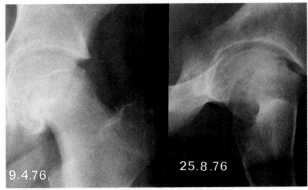

537 This 12-year-old was complaining of discomfort in the hip and limped from time-to-time. An X-ray revealed poor development of the right acetabulum. This was due to a congenital dislocation of the hip that had not been noticed at birth.

538 This rather plump 14-year-old presented with pain in the hips and limping; note the slipped epiphysis, seen best in the lateral view.

Hip Pain

- Transient synovitis (observation and/or irritable hip)
- Bacterial infection
- Avascular necrosis (Perthes' disease)
- Slipped epiphysis
- Protrusio acetabuli
- Arthritis:
    B27 arthropathy
    Other forms of juvenile arthritis
    Rheumatic fever
- Malignancy:
    Local:
        benign (e.g., osteoid osteoma)
        malignant (e.g., Ewing's sarcoma)
    Generalized:
        leukaemia
        neuroblastoma

Vitamin D Metabolic Problems

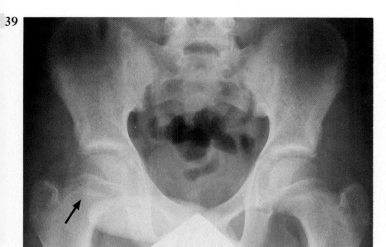

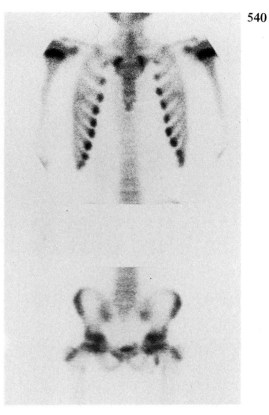

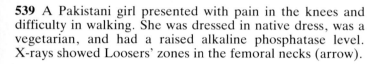

539 A Pakistani girl presented with pain in the knees and difficulty in walking. She was dressed in native dress, was a vegetarian, and had a raised alkaline phosphatase level. X-rays showed Loosers' zones in the femoral necks (arrow).

540 Technetium bone scan of the girl in **539**, which not only showed up her epiphyses, but also Loosers' zones.

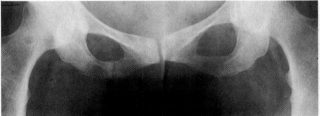

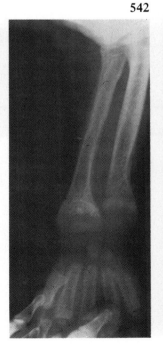

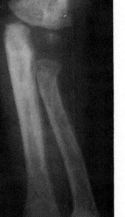

541 Another Pakistani girl who presented with pain in the groin and difficulty in standing. Note Loosers' zones, characteristic of osteomalacia, in the right pubic ramus.

542,543 This 10-month-old baby was brought to hospital because of screaming and dislike of being touched. X-rays revealed gross ricketts. These were actually nutritional, as he lived indoors and had been fed on condensed milk.

Hypermobility

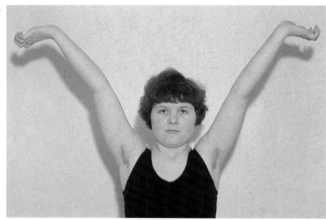

544 This teenager had marked hypermobility at her elbows and wrists. She was a 'sports' girl and presented with traumatic effusions in her knees.

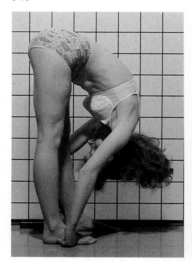

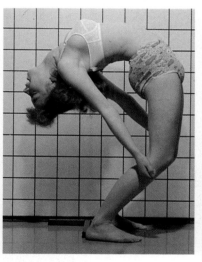

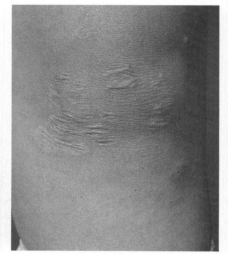

545,546 This girl, who presented with aches and pains in many sites, was noted to be markedly hypermobile, particularly in the spine and hips.

547 Scars of striae associated with Ehlers–Danlos syndrome, particularly Type III, which causes hypermobility, easy bruising and a tendency to aching in the joints.

Multiple Epiphyseal Dysplasia

- Associated with pain and stiffness in the limbs followed by the development of contractures
- The dysplasia most likely to give rise to problems in diagnosis is the tarda form of spondo-epiphyseal dysplasia, which does not usually present until the age of 3 or 4, or even as late as 7 or 8 years

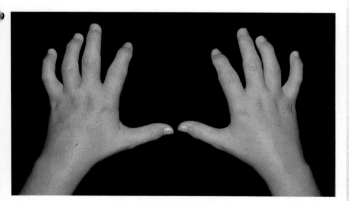

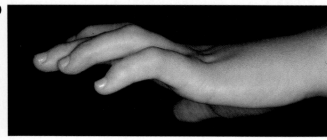

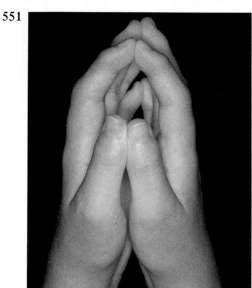

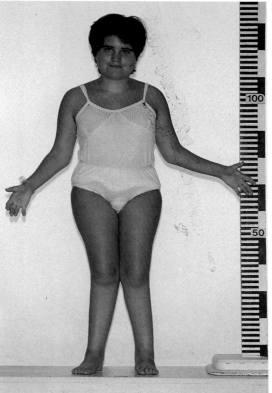

548 This girl, shown here at age 16, presented at the age of 3 with difficulty in climbing up stairs, followed at the age of 5 with difficulty in using her hands.

549 This shows the hands of the girl in **548** with bony enlargement of all the phalangeal joints and a tendency to clawing.

550 In the lateral view of one hand of the girl in **548**, the difficulty in extending the fingers is obvious.

551 The bony enlargement of the thumbs and first metacarpophalangeal joint in the girl in **548**, together with the enlargement of the other joints and the inability to fully extend either hand.

552

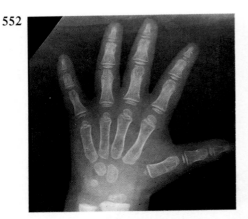

553

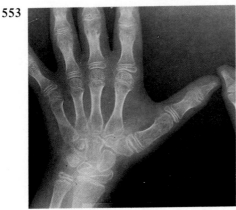

554

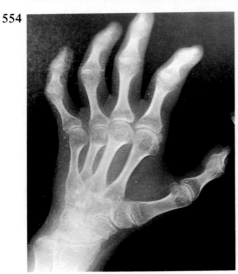

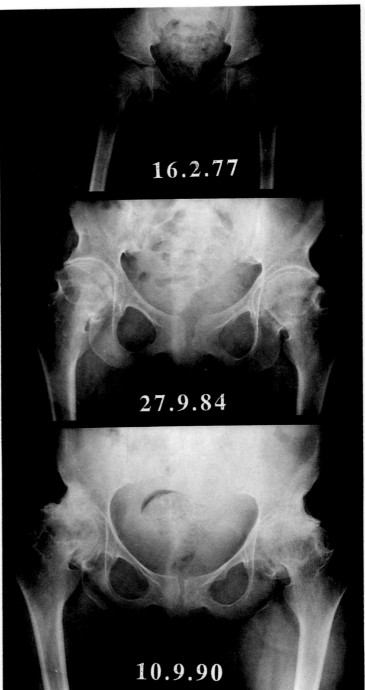

552–554 The progressive radiological changes that have occurred in the girl in **548**, at presentation (**552**), 5 years later (**553**) and at 16 years old (**554**).

555 Sequential hip films from 1977, when the girl in **548** just showed a skeletal dysplasia, to the condition in 1990, at which time she underwent total replacement arthroplasty (she was 18 years old).

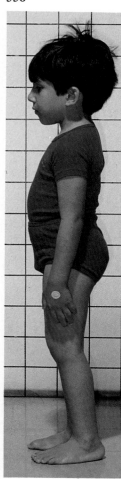
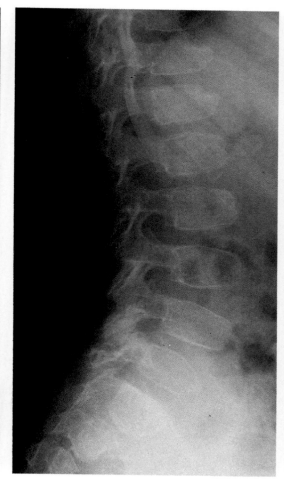
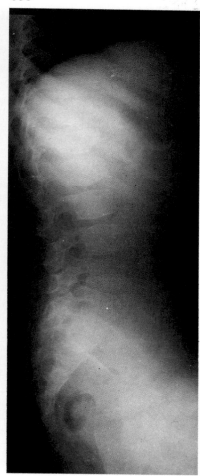

556 This 7-year-old boy presented with a waddling gait and some difficulty in using his hands. The bony enlargement of the hands, together with a normal ESR, suggested an epiphyseal dysplasia.

557 The lateral view of the spine of the boy in **556**; note the anterior indentation of the vertebrae.

558 This shows the vertebrae of the girl in **548**, showing the abnormal shape of the vertebra as she proceeds into adult life. Symptoms of spinal stenosis have been seen in some of our patients.

559 Late cervical spine which is mimicking juvenile arthritis. Note the odontoid process is tending to go forward and the unusual shape of the vertebra in an 18-year-old.

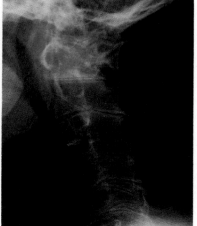

559

Mucopolysaccharidoses

- These inborn errors of mucopolysaccharide metabolism are associated with a skeletal dysplasia, which can present as a joint problem, particularly clawing of the hands
- The dysplasia most likely to be confused with juvenile chronic arthritis is Scheie's, as the progressive stiffening of the joints does not begin until about the age of 4 or 5. There is no failure of growth, and a normal facies and mentality are present

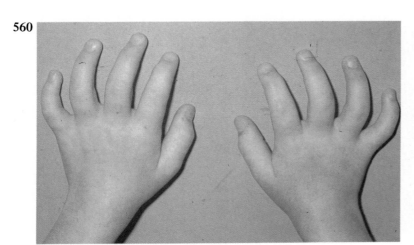

560 A 5-year-old girl presented with difficulty in using her hands and was found to have clawing and also stiffness of the shoulders, with some limitation of movement of the hips, knees and elbows. A tentative diagnosis of juvenile chronic arthritis (polyarticular type) was made, but there was no soft-tissue swelling of the joints and her ESR was normal. An excess of dermatan sulphate was found in the urine.

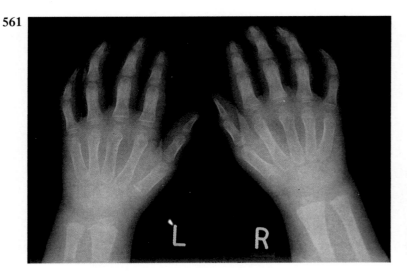

561 X-ray of the hands of a 7-year-old suffering from Scheie's syndrome, in which clawing of the hands is obvious. Apart from osteoporosis, there are no significant radiological changes. (Courtesy of Prof. E.G.L. Bywaters, UK.)

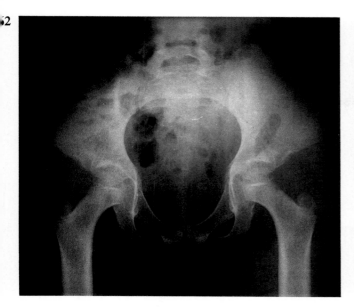

562 Skeletal dysostosis in Hurler's syndrome, showing abnormality of the hip bone texture and development.

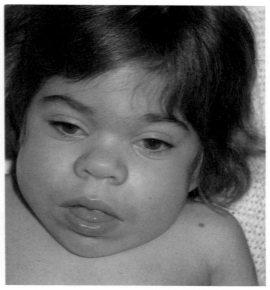

563 Typical facies of Hurler's syndrome.

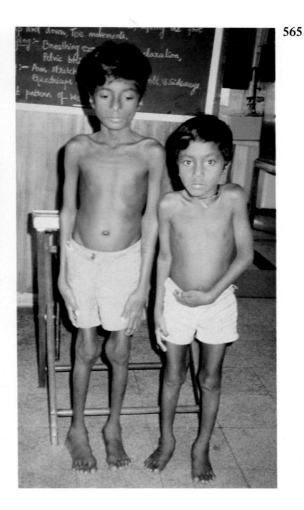

564 This 11-year-old was stunted in overall growth, with small limbs and a loss of function. He was diagnosed as Hunter's syndrome with increased excretion of dermatan sulphate and heparin sulphate. Note the skeletal dysostosis present in the wrists and interphalangeal joints. (Courtesy of Prof. E.G.L. Bywaters, UK.)

565 Cousins with Morquio–Brailsford disease. (Courtesy of Prof. Chanderasaki, India.)

Mucolipidoses

- Mucolipidosis Type III, which is sometimes known as pseudo-Hurler's polydystrophy, is the one most likely to be confused with juvenile arthritis, as restriction of joint mobility does not usually become apparent until the second or third year of life.
- Biochemically, there is a deficiency in Glc Nac P-transferase in fibroblasts and leucocytes

566

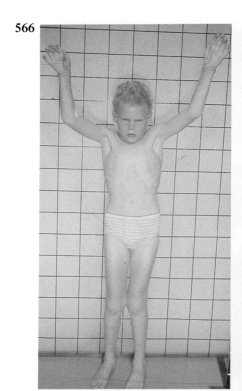

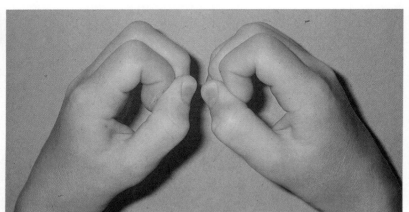

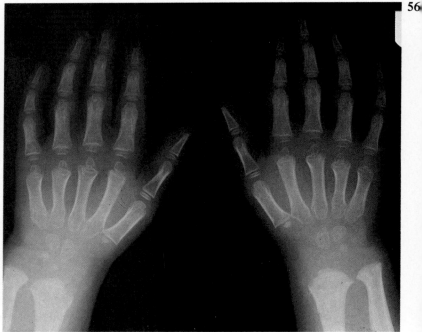

566 This boy presented at the age of 3 with a slight difficulty in making a fist. This became progressively worse and he was found to have marked difficulty in elevating the shoulders.

567 This shows the marked thickening of soft tissues on the palmar aspect of the hand, with difficulty in pinching, in the boy in **566**.

568 X-rays of another child who presented with difficulty in using her hands at 6 years of age. Note the unusual ends to the radius and ulnar, as well as changes in the small bones of the hands.

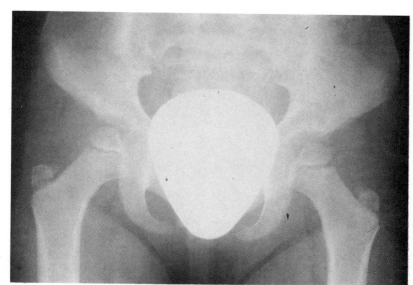

569 X-ray of the pelvis of the case in **568**, showing marked dysplasia of the hips.

Sphingolipidoses

Farber's lipogranulomatosis

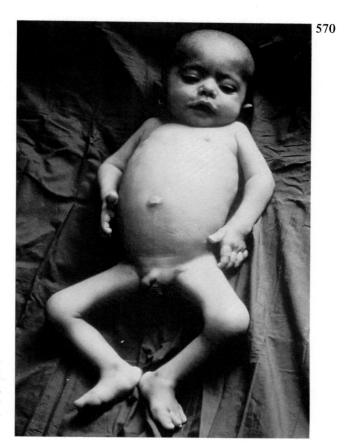

570 This Pakistan baby was extremely irritable. He had a history of masses around the joints, followed by the development of the contractures of the hips and knees shown here. As he cried he was very husky and his mental development was below normal. He had a deficiency of acid ceramidase.

571

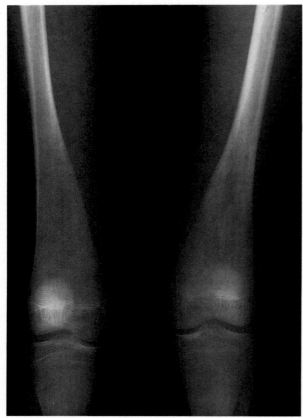

571 Gaucher's disease Type III frequently presents as a polyarthralgia due to infiltration of the marrow of the subchondral bone, in turn due to the accumulation of glucosyl ceramide as a result of deficiency in acid glucosidase. This X-ray shows the classic Erlenmeyer's flask deformities of the lower femurs.

572

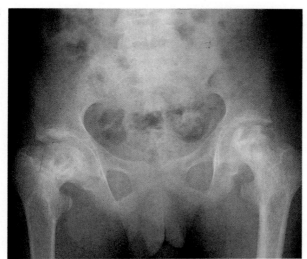

572 X-ray of the pelvis showing short femoral necks with obvious infiltration and deformed femoral heads.

Sarcoidosis

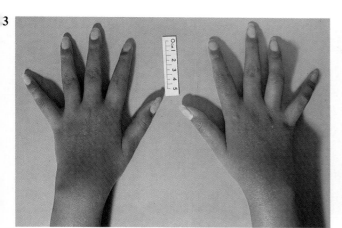

573 Swelling of the wrists in a 5-year-old.

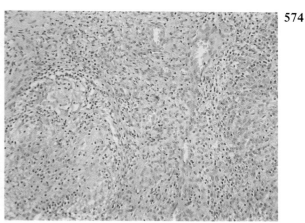

574 Biopsy of a synovial membrane, showing noncaseating granuloma.

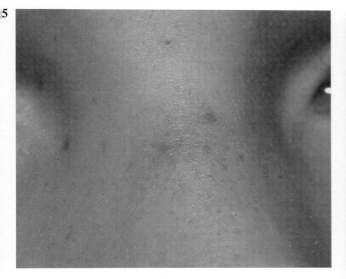

575 Rash on the nose of a 3-year-old who presented with boggy swollen knees.

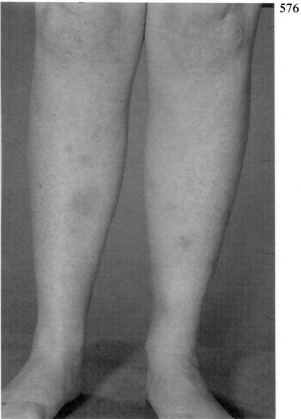

576 A 13-year-old Caucasian who presented with erythema nodosum.

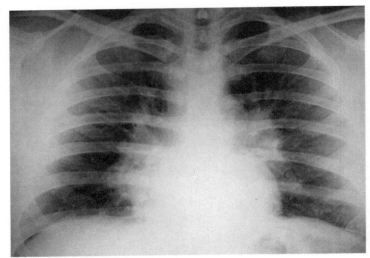

577 Chest X-ray of the case shown in **576**, indicating bilateral lymphadenopathy.

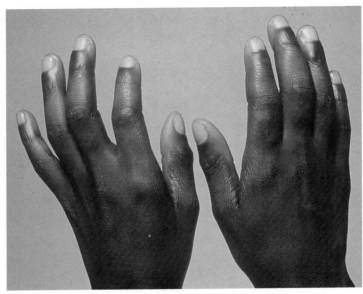

578 Bony enlargement led to apparent flexion contractures at the proximal inter-phalangeal joints in this teenage boy.

Panniculitis

- Characterized by inflammation of fatty tissues
- Does not represent a single disease
- Crops of painful subcutaneous nodules, thighs, legs, abdomen and arms, which may leave pigmented depressions
- Can be associated with fever and arthralgia

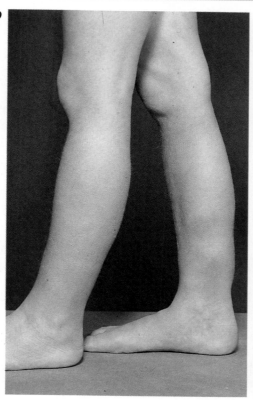

579

579 Note the large lesions mimicking erythema nodosum, but occurring towards the back of the leg.

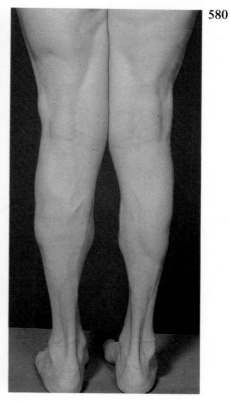

580

580 Posterior view of the legs of a girl who has had recurrent lesions; note the atrophy of fat in the lower part.

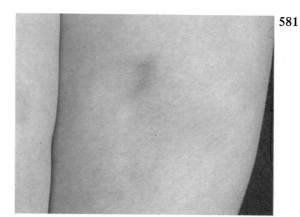

581

581 Close-up of a lesion on the upper thigh of the girl in **580**.

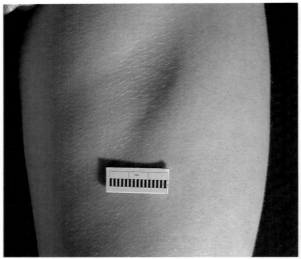

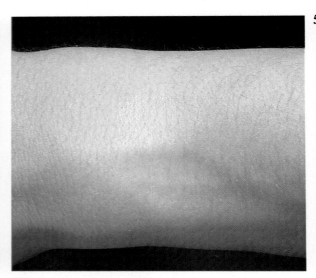

582 Close-up of the indentation left as panniculitis subsided in another girl.

583 Scarring from a lesion in the arm.

Benign Rheumatoid Nodules

- Characterized by subcutaneous nodules, usually affecting the pre-tibial area, but they can also occur on the occiput, elbows and forearms, and paraspinally

- Can be associated with granuloma annulare
- Not associated with the later development of arthritis or with rheumatoid factor

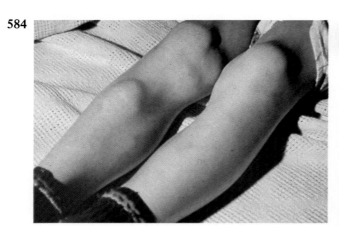

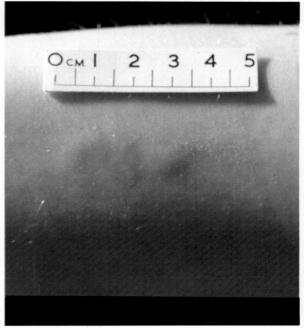

584 Benign rheumatoid nodules of 5 months' duration in a 7-year-old boy who was otherwise healthy. The nodules were non-tendor, and subsequently regressed, leaving no residual marks (Simons and Schaller, 1975).

585 Pseudo-rheumatoid nodules in the pre-tibial area in a 9-year-old girl.

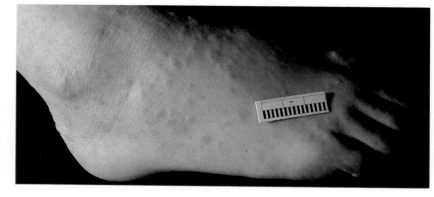

586 Typical granuloma annulare with the nodules in the skin. Histologically, these are composed of fibrinoid necrotic areas surrounded by palisades of histocytes and mononuclear cells.

Other Soft-Tissue Lesions

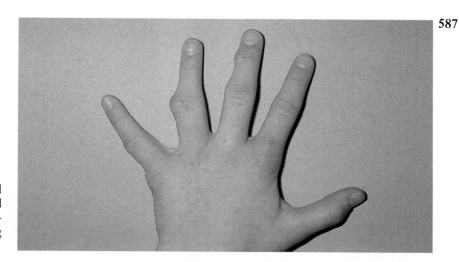

587 Fibromata over proximal interphalangeal joints 4 and (lesser) 3, and terminal interphalangeal joint 3 mimicking soft-tissue swelling.

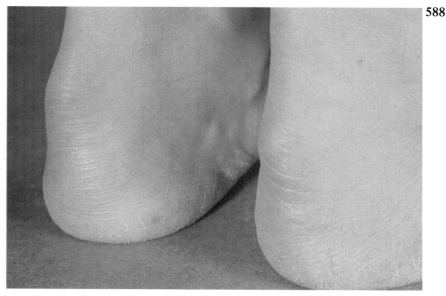

588 This 12-year-old presented with discomfort in the heels and nodules over the metacarpophalangeal joints, due to cholesterol deposits. He had suffered an episode of arthritis in the ankles and wrists, which lasted for a few days. His plasma cholesterol was high and he had a slightly raised ESR. Thus, he belonged to hypercholesterolaemia type II and was homozygous.

Chronic Infantile Neurological and Articular Syndrome (CINCA) – Infantile Onset Multisystem Inflammatory Disease (IOMID)

- Often premature
- Rash, urticarial, blotchy (neonatal)
- Hepatosplenomegaly, lymphadenopathy
- Fever
- ESR rises, WBC rises, haemoglobin level falls
- Arthropathy in the large joints, particularly the knees, from 1 year or more
- Chronic neurological involvement

- Also the following can occur:
  growth retardation
  delayed closure anterior fontanelle
  eye lesions
  deafness
  dental anomalies
  progeria hands and feet
  mental retardation

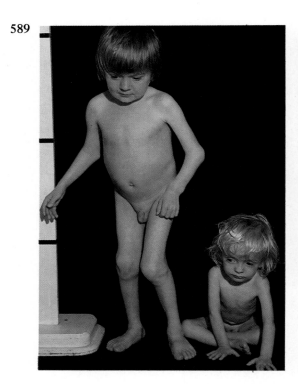

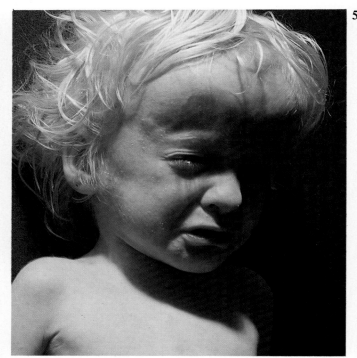

589 Two siblings with the CINCA syndrome. Note the older boy is standing, but with flexed knees, and the 2-year-old girl cannot stand.

590 Close-up of the face of the girl in **589**, showing the high prominent forehead; the anterior fontanelle remained open until she was 5 years old.

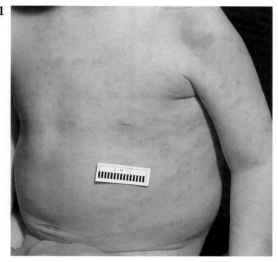

591 Rash of the girl in **589** mimicking systemic juvenile arthritis, but itchy, larger and present all the time.

592 Rash on another boy which was even more marked and had an urticarial element, and at times became extremely red after scratching.

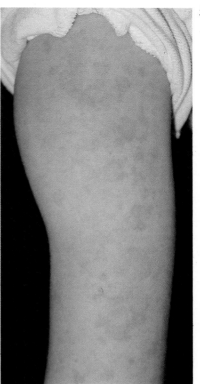

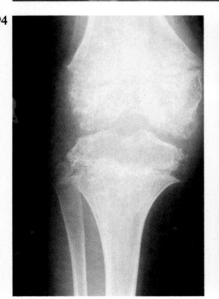

593 X-ray of the knees of the brother (RB) and sister (CB) shown in **589**. Note the large patellae and the changes in epiphyses, the boy's more advanced than the girl's, that are taking place.

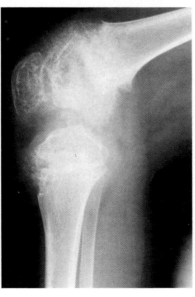

594,595 Posterio-anterior and lateral X-rays of the knee of the boy in **589**, showing the marked epiphyseal changes and the large patella.

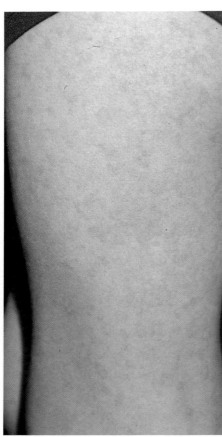

596 Rash in another child which tends to mimic erythema multiforme.

597 Massive enlargement of the patellae clinically in another boy also with profuse rash.

598 Another child with CINCA syndrome, who was first noted to have a rash when she was in an incubator after a premature birth. Although she appeared to be thriving, she continued to have rashes and, at about 7 months, she was noted to be anaemic and had hepatosplenomegaly. At the age of 1 year she was not walking properly and her knee swelling was first noted. She continued to have bouts of synovitis over many years, fairly well controlled by corticosteroids, but being exacerbated with every intercurrent infection.

599 X-ray of an elbow in the boy in **589**, showing progressive changes in the epiphyseal development over a 1-year period.

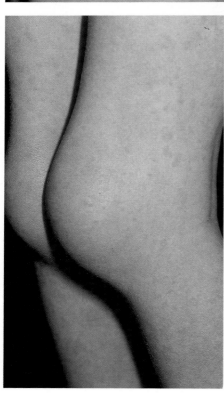

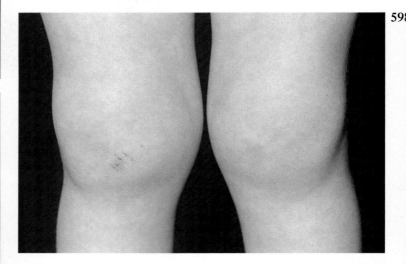

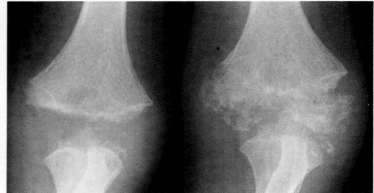

Variant of CINCA (IOMID)

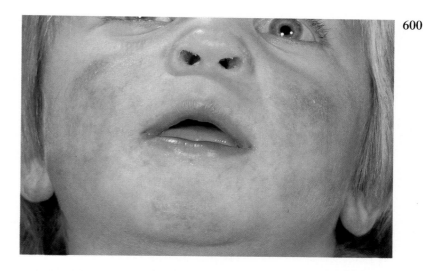

600,601 This boy failed to thrive from the age of 7 months and developed a rash which was sometimes urticarial and at other times eczematous. Over the next few months he became progressively anaemic and had a rising ESR, refused to make any attempt to stand and developed contractures at the hips and knees and fingers. Because of the high ESR and poor haemoglobin and some fever, he was put onto corticosteroids with some benefit as regards the lower limbs, but he continued to have severe contractures of his fingers (**601**).

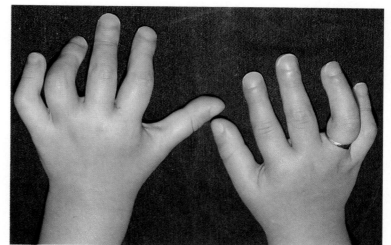

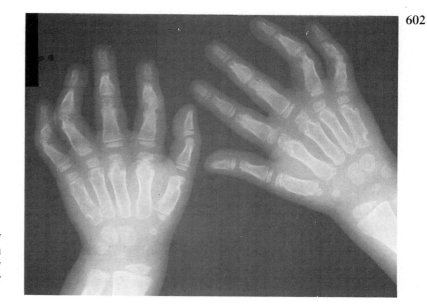

602 X-rays of the hands of the boy in **600** and **601**, showing absorption of the terminal phalanges, with bony changes in some of the other phalanges.

Acro-osteolysis

● May be hereditary or idiopathic; the latter is frequently associated with the later development of a progressive renal lesion

603

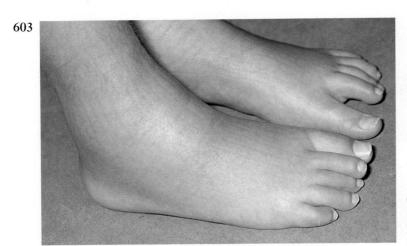

603 This 4-year-old presented as limping and complained of pain in her feet. She was found to have swelling. The ESR was normal, as was the X-ray.

604 **605**

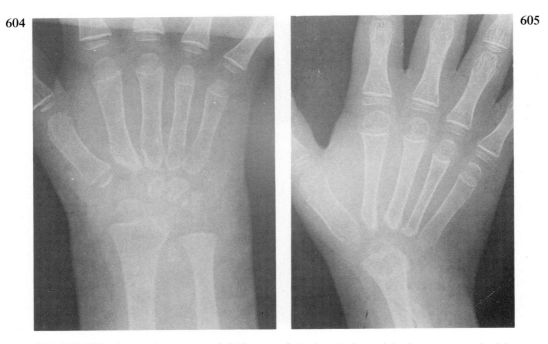

604,605 This shows the sequential X-rays of the hands in a girl who presented with swelling of the wrists when 18 months old. A year later, pencilling of the base of the metacarpals, particularly 2, had occurred, as had shortening of the ulnar (**604**). A sequential X-ray 2¼ years later shows there has been complete loss of carpal bones and change in the shape of the radius and the ulnar (**605**).

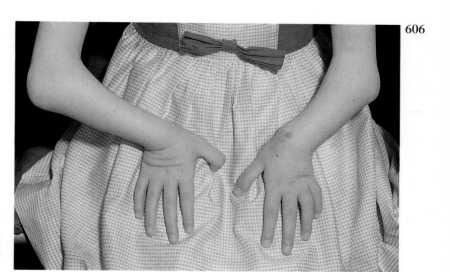

606 Appearance of the hands and wrists of the patient in **604**, 6 years into the disease.

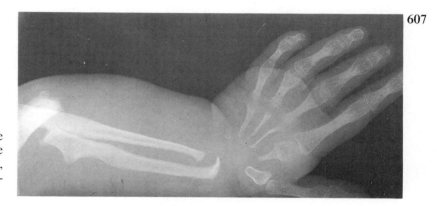

607 X-rays taken at the same time as **606**, showing further loss of bone in the metacarpi, radius and ulna, and that the elbow has begun to disintegrate.

Pachydermoperiostitis

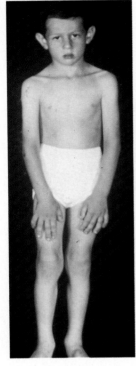

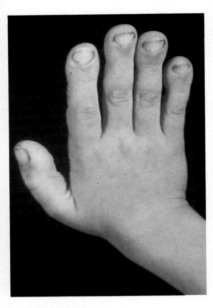

608 Young boy presenting with swollen knees; note the normal facies at this age.

609 Spatula-shaped hand with finger clubbing from the patient in **608**.

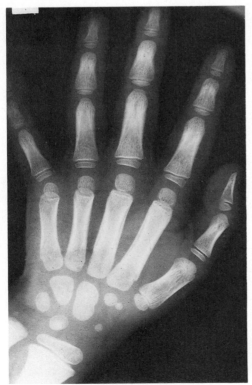

610 X-ray of a hand similar to that in **609**, showing periostitis along the radius and metacarpophalangeal joints.

Reflex Dystrophy

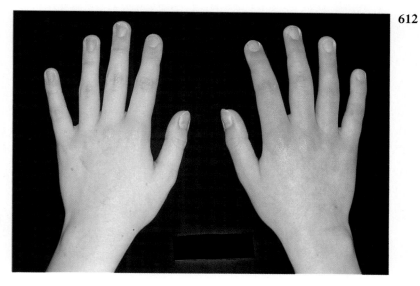

611

611 This girl presented with a painful swollen hand which proved to be oedematous. She had a history of a fall and a fractured humerus. This is a reflex dystrophy in a girl who was frightened to report her initial injury to her family (there was much family tension).

612

612 Marked changes in the colour of the hands. This boy was refusing to use the hand at all. Diagnosis of reflex dystrophy was made and he responded to a guanethidine block.

Trichorhinophalangeal Dysplasia

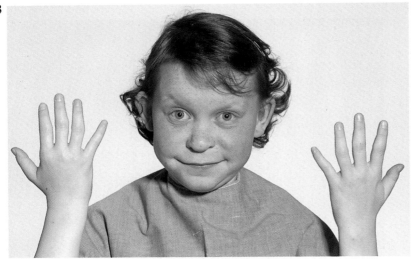

613 Trichorhinophalangeal dysplasia is characterized by enlargement of the interphalangeal joints. Note the appearance of the nose and hyperplastic nares and large ears. (Courtesy of Dr A. Craft, UK.)

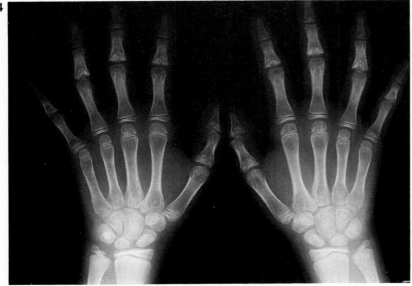

614 X-ray showing coning of epiphyses, particularly of the proximal intephalangeal joints and alteration in shape of the base of the proximal phalangeal joints. (Courtesy of Dr A. Craft, UK.)

Arthrogryphosis

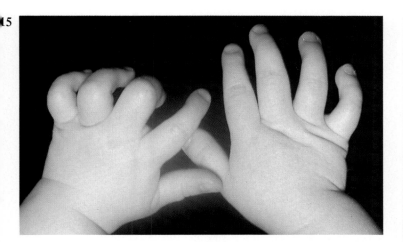

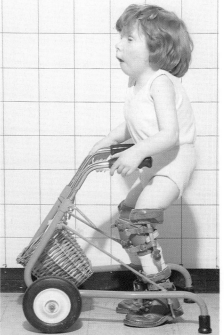

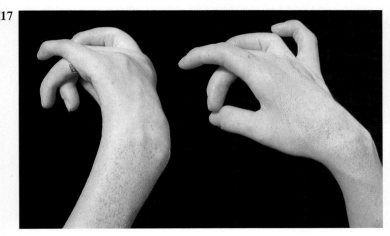

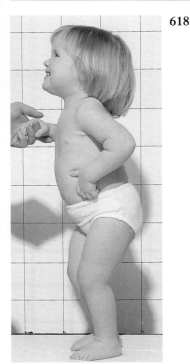

615 Contractures of the proximal interphalangeal joints in a young child with arthrogryphosis.

616 Note the flexed elbows and, even with splints, this child's knees cannot be straightened. She needs a walker in order to move.

617 This teenager had received no physiotherapy or splinting for her condition. Note the fixed wrists, the hyperextended metacarpophalangeal joints and the flexed proximal interphalangeal joints.

618 This plump baby shows fixed-flexion contractures of the elbows, wrists, hips and knees. Her plumpness makes it difficult to appreciate that she has really no muscle to palpate underneath.

Note that in some 40% of children only the lower limbs are affected and in 10% only the upper limbs.

Unusual Problems

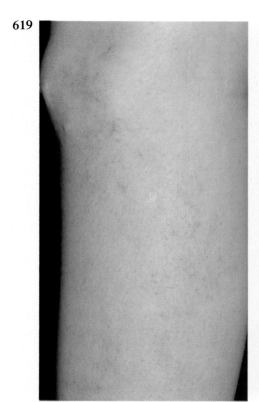

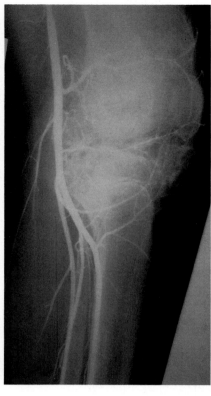

619 Recurrent bleeding into the knee in a girl, aged 10 in this illustration, whose symptoms had commenced at the age of 3. Note the vascular malformation along the leg.

620 Arteriography of **619**, showing communication of the cutaneous lesion with the vessels of the synovial lining.

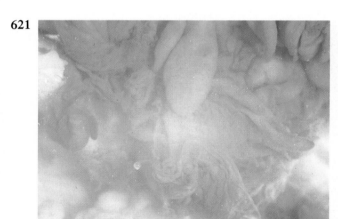

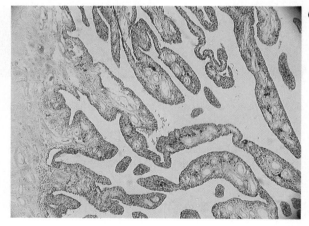

621 Appearances of pigmented villonodular synovitis in a teenager who presented with recurrent haemarthrosis in a knee which later remained persistently swollen.

622 Histology from the case in **621**, showing iron deposition in the villous fronds.

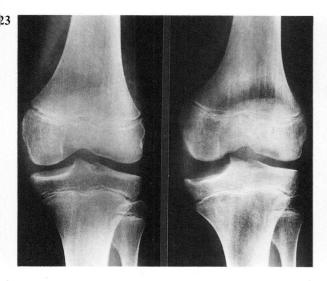 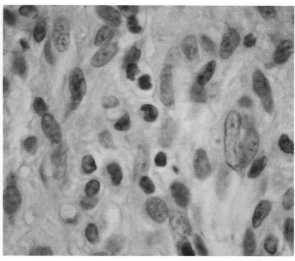

623,624 Persistent swelling of the knee (**623**) in a teenager with general malaise and raised ESR. Histology of the knee (**624**) revealed synovioma, which is an excessively rare condition in both children and adults.

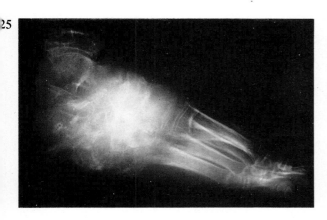

25

625 Radiograph of the ankle and foot of a teenager who had suffered a swollen painful foot for several months, and who had been treated for pauci-articular juvenile rheumatic arthritis. The radiograph shows the obvious changes of a bone tumour, an osteoblastoma which was responsible for all of the physical findings and complaints.

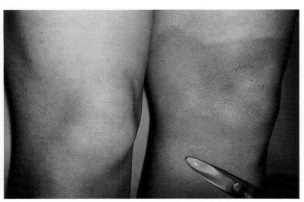

26

626 Acute swelling of the knee, associated with fever and abdominal pain, which commenced at age 6 years in a Turkish child. Episodes of arthritis resolved in about 3 weeks. The synovial fluid showed a polymorphonuclear cytosis reaction. (Courtesy of Dr H. Ozdogan, Turkey.)

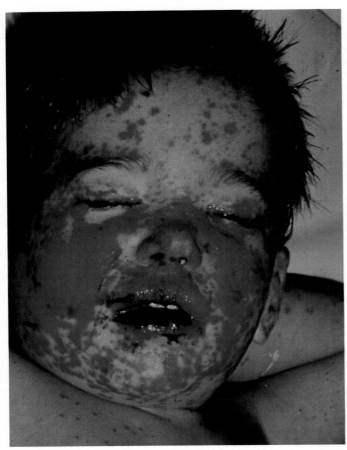

627 Typical oral, nasal, conjunctival and cutaneous manifestations of severe Stevens–Johnson syndrome. (From Behrman and Vaughan, 1987; courtesy of W.B. Saunders, USA.)

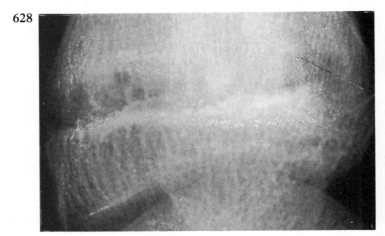

628 X-ray of ankle from a 12-year-old girl who presented with a painful swelling of an ankle followed by a knee and then the other ankle. Full investigations were undertaken with the only abnormality being a raised ESR and changes on the X-rays, as shown here, which mimicked the deposition seen in leukaemia. The bone marrow was normal and a biopsy of the affected area showed no evidence of infection. It was concluded that as she had three sites, and then a further two developed, this was chronic focal sterile osteomyelitis.

629 This 5-year-old girl presented with a painful hip, followed by severe pain in her back, which caused a vertebra to collapse; note the changes below the epiphysis in the hips. To rule out eosinophilic granuloma, a biopsy was undertaken. Non-specific granulation tissue was detected for which no cause could be found. She eventually healed spontaneously in both affected sites after approximately a year.

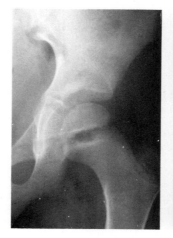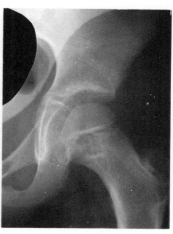

Limb pains with no organic basis (Apley, 1976)

- Both sexes
- 6–13 years
- Predominantly lower limbs
- Can be only nocturnal
- No deterioration in general health
- Emotional disturbances common
- Headache and/or abdominal pain in two-fifths of cases
- Family history common

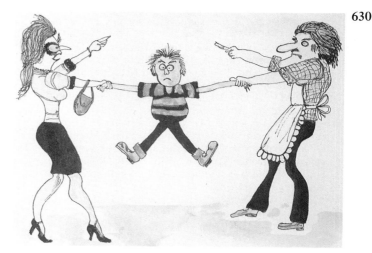

630 A cartoon representing recurrent limb pain, drawn by a child in a household where there was considerable family tension.

Children at Risk for HIV Infection

- Children of HIV infected mothers
- Adolescents infected by sexual intercourse
- Adolescents infected by intravenous drug abuse
- Haemophiliacs
- Can present as muscle, skin or joint problems
- Children may present as PUO accompanied by organomegaly and other quasi-rheumatic complaints
- Generalized lymphadenopathy
- Thrombocytopenia

REFERENCES

American College of Rheumatology (1990), Criteria for the Classification of Vasculitis, *Arthritis and Rheumatism*, **33**, 1065–1136.

Ansell, B.M. (1990), Classification and a Nomenclature, *Paediatric Rheumatology Update*, Oxford University Press, pp 3–5.

Ansell, B.M. (1988), Scleroderma in Childhood, In *Systemic Sclerosis (Scleroderma)*, Jayson, M.V. and Black, C.M. (Eds), Wiley, Bristol, pp 319–330.

Apley, J. (1976), Limb Pain with no Organic Disease, *Clinical Rheumatic Disorders*, **2**, 487–491.

Behrman, R.E. and Vaughan, V.C., III, *Nelson Textbook of Pediatrics*, W.B. Saunders, Philadelphia.

Bywaters, E.G.L. (1977), The History of Paediatric Rheumatology, *Arthritis and Rheumatism*, **20** (Suppl. 2), 145–152.

Cassidy, J.T., Levinson, J.E., and Brewer, E.J. (1989), The Development of Classification Criteria for Children with Juvenile Rheumatoid Arthritis, *Bulletin on the Rheumatic Diseases*, **38**, 1–7.

Pope, R.M. (1989), Rheumatic Fever in the 1980s, *Bulletin on the Rheumatic Diseases*, **38**(3), 1–8.

Prieur, A.M., Ansell, B.M., Bardfield, R. *et al.* (1990), Is Onset Type Evaluated During the First 3 Months of Disease Satisfactory for Defining the Subgroups of Juvenile Chronic Arthritis? A EULAR Cooperative Study (1983–1986), *Clinical and Experimental Rheumatology*, **8**, 321–325.

Savage, C.O.S., Winearls, C.G., Jones, S., Marshall, P.D., and Lockwood, C.M. (1987), Prospective Study of Radio-Immunoassay for Antibodies against Neutrophil Cytoplasm in the Diagnosis of Systemic Vasculitis, *Lancet*, **i**, 1389–1393.

Shulman, S.T. (Ed.) *et al.* (1989), Management of Kawasaki Syndrome: A Consensus Statement Prepared by North American Participants of the Third International Kawasaki Disease Symposium, Tokyo, Japan, December, 1988, *Paediatric Infectious Diseases Journal*, **8**, 663–665.

Simons, F.E.R. and Schaller, J.G. (1975), Benign Rheumatoid Arthritis, *Pediatrics*, **56**, 29–33.

Southwood, T.R., Petty, R.E., Malleson, P.N., Delgardo, E.A., Hunt, D.W.C., Wood, B., and Schroeder, M.L. (1989), Psoriatic Arthritis in Children, *Arthritis and Rheumatism*, **32**, 1007–1013.

Stollerman, C.H., Markowitz, M., Taranta, A., Wanamakter, L.W., and Whittlemore, R. (1965), Jone's Criteria (Revised) for Guidance in the Diagnosis of Rheumatic Fever, *Circulation*, **32**, 664–668.

Suzuki, A., Tizard, E.J., Gooch, V., *et al.* (1990), Kawasaki Disease: Echocardiographic Features in 91 Cases Presenting in the United Kingdom, *Archives of Disease in Childhood*, **1990**, 1142–1146.

Tan, E.M., Cohen, A.S., Fries, J.F., *et al.* (1982), The 1982 Revised Criteria for the Classification of Systemic Lupus Erythematosus, *Arthritis and Rheumatism*, **25**, 1127–1128.

FURTHER READING

Ansell, B.M. (1980), *Rheumatic Disorders in Childhood*, Butterworths, London.

Beighton, P., Grahame, R., and Bird, H. (1989), *Hypermobility of Joints*, 2nd edn, Springer, Verlag, Berlin.

Cassidy, J.T. and Petty, R. (1990), *Textbook of Paediatric Rheumatology*, 2nd edn, Churchill Livingstone, Edinburgh.

Dubowitz, V. (1989), *A Colour Atlas of Muscular Disorders in Childhood*, Wolfe Publishing Ltd, London.

Jacobs, J.C. (1982), *Paediatric Rheumatology for the Practitioner*, Springer Verlag, Berlin.

Schaller, J.G. and Hanson, V. (1977), Proceedings of the First American Rheumatism Association Conference of the Rheumatic Diseases of Childhood, *Arthritis and Rheumatism*, **20** (Suppl. 2), 145–636.

Williams, G.F. (1981), *Children with Chronic Arthritis*, PSG Publishing.

Woo, P., White, P., and Ansell, B.M. (1990), *Update in Paediatric Rheumatology*, Oxford University Press.

Wynne-Davies, R., Hall, C.M., and Apley, A.G. (1985), *Atlas of Skeletal Dysplasias*, Churchill Livingstone, Edinburgh.

INDEX